THE ACCENT METHOD OF VOICE THERAPY

M. Nasser Kotby, M.D.
Professor and Chairperson
Unit of Phoniatrics and Communicative Disorders
Faculty of Medicine
Ain Shams University
Cairo, Egypt

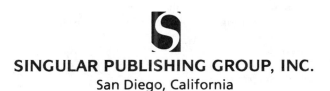

SINGULAR PUBLISHING GROUP, INC.
San Diego, California

Singular Publishing Group, Inc.
4284 41st Street
San Diego, California 92105-1197

© 1995 by Singular Publishing Group, Inc.

Typeset in 10/12 Century Schoolbook by So Cal Graphics
Printed in the United States of America by McNaughton & Gunn

Library of Congress Cataloging-in-Publication Data

Kotby, M. Nasser.
    The accent method of voice therapy / M. Nasser Kotby.
      p. cm.
    Includes bibliographical references and index.
    ISBN 1-56593-090-8
    1. Voice of disorders—Treatment.   I. Title.
    [DNLM: 1. Voice Disorders—therapy   WV 500 K87a 1994]
  RF540.K68   1994
  616.85'506—dc20
  DNLM/DLC
  for Library of Congress   94-35258
                                         CIP

THE ACCENT METHOD OF VOICE THERAPY

CONTENTS

PREFACE

∎

In the summer of 1972, I attended an intensive course on the Accent Method (AM) given by Svend Smith, himself. I returned from the course full of enthusiasm and began to apply the Accent Method (AM) in Sweden, where I was studying phoniatrics. Since then, I have applied this method successfully to a large number of voice patients with a variety of vocal pathologies. The ethnicity of my patients has ranged from Europeans and Egyptians to Middle Easterners and Japanese.

During the years of clinical work, many questions have arisen about the Accent Method (AM). These were discussed with Svend Smith personally and with some of his disciples, such as Arthur and Ulla Boberg from Denmark and Bibi Fex from Sweden, who have actively helped the Ain Shams University Phoniatrics and Logopedics Unit by lectures, demonstration, and clinical application of the Accent Method (AM). This has added a great deal to the education of my junior colleagues, as well as the broadening of my own experience in that field. This close contact and exchange of information fortunately fruitfully continues.

In presenting the Accent Method (AM) of voice therapy in this book, I first review the pathophysiological model of voice disorders and the etiological classification of these disorders. This is a necessary prerequisite to understanding the theory and indications and uses of the Accent Method (AM) of voice therapy. The importance of a detailed assessment of voice production before determining a management plan is stressed throughout the text. An outline of a comprehensive assessment protocol is provided in Appendix 1. Alternative management strategies are briefly summarized to allow readers to put the Accent Method (AM) in perspective relative to other available treatments.

The introductory chapters are followed by a detailed description of the rationale and methodology of the Accent Method (AM). The various considerations for the practical application of the Accent Method (AM) are presented. An audiotape with a sample of the basic accent exercises provides a practical demonstration for help in self-teaching and in giving readers a deeper perspective. The audiotape is probably more practical and effective than a videotape. The latter is, however, available on request.

ACKNOWLEDGMENTS

■

I would like to express my sincere thanks to my colleagues in the Department of Otolaryngology (Dr. Ali G. Abd El-Rahman) and in the Unit of Phoniatrics and Logopedics (Drs. Samia Bassiouny, Marwa Saleh, Aliaa Khidr, Mona Hegazi, Nirvana Gamal, and Amal Sayed), Faculty of Medicine, Ain Shams University for the great efforts and the indispensable assistance they have offered to make this work a reality.

INTRODUCTION

■

Communication disorders have a long history. Ancient Egyptian medicine includes descriptions of cases including speech problems, but does not offer any suggestion for treatment (E. Smith Surgical Papyrus, Case 20, cited in Brested, 1930).

Later, Greek medicinal scholars enhanced our knowledge by identifying the clinical importance of voice change as a presenting symptom of systemic diseases (Hippocrates, ca 460–377 B.C.E., as cited in Stevenson & Guthrie, 1949). Approximately 600 years later, Galen (ca 130–200 C.E., as cited in Stevenson & Guthrie, 1949), described the laryngeal mechanism, illustrating laryngeal cartilages and muscles, plus their innervation by the recurrent laryngeal nerve. He presented conclusive evidence that the larynx is the voice source. Through the teaching and practices of Demosthenes (ca 384–322 B.C.E.), a major step in the field of voice therapy was achieved. Demosthenes' sophisticated methods for the labeling of breathing and articulatory production aimed at improving voice and speech (Plutarkhos, 1947) served as a cornerstone for subsequent development of what we currently call behavioral management.

The evolution of voice treatment included many texts written before the Middle Ages. Al-Razy (Latin: Rhazes) (865–925 C.E., as cited in Hussein & Al Okbi, 1977), in his comprehensive clinical book of medicine *Al-Hawi* (known through its Latin translation, *Continens*), gave a detailed description of voice disorders, principles of vocal hygiene, and voice training exercises. Ibn Sina (Latin: Avicenna) (980–1037 C.E.) in his textbook of medicine *Al Qanun*, elaborated on Al-Razy's teaching about voice disorders and their management. Most noteworthy were his elaborate treatises on the laryngeal anatomy. Another medical author from Cairo, Ibn Al-Nafis (1288 C.E.), who was the first to discover and describe pulmonary circulation, recommended a vocal hygiene program for patients with voice disorders that is similar to programs used today.

The development in medical sciences during the European Renaissance, centered round the fifteenth and sixteenth centuries, added crucial information about laryngeal structure and function (Vesalius, 1542 C.E., as cited in Stevenson & Guthrie, 1949). There was, however, no particular description of management of voice disorders nor voice therapy.

The nineteenth century has witnessed the onset of a discipline of clinical laryngology based not only on astute clinical observation but also on results of numerous experiments. Much of this was made possible by visualization of the larynx first accomplished by Manuel Garcia (1855), who used a small mirror in the back of the throat, with a sunlight light. This procedure opened the way for the development of modern laryngology. Since then, several great men and women have devoted their scientific careers to enhance our knowledge about the larynx and voice production.

The need for knowledge about voice therapy resulted from the recognition of a special category of voice disorders for which the laryngologist could not find an organic cause of the disorder that could be treated with surgery. The laryngologist realized that usual surgical and pharmacological procedures were of little use in the management of these cases. Adjustments of the patients' vocal habits were thought to be an alternative to surgical and pharmacological treatment, but little was known about how to accomplish the desired change. This led to the emergence of the need for voice therapy.

During the nineteenth and early twentieth centuries, articles and texts were primarily directed toward training the singing voice. The emergence and development of voice therapy for the management of pathological conditions of the speaking voice occurred much later. Few phoniatricians and logopedists (speech pathologists), described training programs for the speaking voice based on their empirical clinical findings. The treatment programs included vocal hygiene and voice drills. These drills focused on specific parts of the speaking apparatus such as the diaphragm, jaw, and throat. The "teacher" was the model and relied heavily on his or her dominant character (Murphy, 1964).

As information accumulated from scientific and clinical laryngology, speech pathology, and phoniatrics, new voice therapy techniques with a physiological rationale were employed to correct the disordered speaking voice. These techniques were already in practice in the 1920s and the 1930s in the leading phoniatric centers of Europe (Forchhammer, 1974; Froeschels, 1932; Gutzmann, 1910 [as cited in Brodnitz, 1971]). Similarly in the United States of America, the works of Van Riper (1939) and others established voice therapy as a scientific clinical practice in the domain of speech pathology.

Since those days, throughout the world several pioneers have described and published their methods of voice therapy (Boone, 1971; Froeschels, 1952; Smith & Thyme, 1978; Weiss, 1955). Not surprisingly, the principles on which these methods (varied as they are) were often influenced by the particular belief (bias) of the clinician concerning laryngeal physiology, structure, and pathology.

It is generally believed that a lot of work is still needed in the field of voice therapy to elucidate the precise scientific rationale for each method of therapy and the therapeutic efficacy of these methods.

REFERENCES

Boone, D. R. (1971). *The voice and voice therapy* (1st ed.), Englewood Cliffs, NJ: Prentice-Hall.

Brested, J. H. (Ed.). (1930). *Edwin Smith surgical papyrus*. Chicago: University of Chicago Press.

Brodnitz, F. S. (1971). *Vocal rehabilitation* (4th ed.). Rochester, MN: American Academy of Ophthalmology and Otolaryngology.

Forchhammer, E. (1974). *Stemmens funktioner of fejlfunktioner*. Copenhagen: Munksgaard.

Froeschels, E. (1932). Über eine neue Behandlungsmethode der Stimmstörungen bei einseitiger Rekurrensslahmung. *Mschr. Ohrenheilk.*, *66*, 1316.

Froeschels, E. (1952). Chewing method as therapy. A discussion with some philosophical conclusions. *Archives of Otolaryngology*, *56*, 427.

Garcia, M. (1855). Physiological observations on the human voice. *Proceedings of the Royal Society, London*, 399.

Hussein, M. K., & Al Okbi, A. (1977). *Teb Al Razi*. Cairo, Egypt: Dar Al Shorouk.

Ibn Al Nafis, A. (1288). *Sharh tashrih al qanun*, makhtout (manuscript) number 3130. Cairo: Dar Al Kotob.

Ibn Sina, A. A. (1294h). *Al quanon fi al tib*. Cairo: Halabi Publisher (Boulaqe edition).

Murphy, A. T. (1964). *Functional voice disorders*. Englewood Cliffs, NJ: Prentice-Hall, Inc.

Plutarkhos. (1947). *Levnadsteckningar över berömda Greker och Romare* [transl. C. Theander, I. Harrie, & H. Bergstedt]. Stockholm: Bokforlaget Natur och kutur.

Smith, S., & Thyme, K. (1978). *Accentmetoden*. Herning: Special Paedagogisk Forlag.

Stevenson, S., & Guthrie, D. (1949). *A history of otolaryngology*. Edinburgh: E. & S. Livingstone.

Van Riper, C. (1939). *Speech correction principles and methods* (1st ed.). London: Constable and Company Ltd.

Weiss, D. A. (1955). The psychological relations towards own voice. *Folia Phoniatrica* (Basel), 7, 209.

CHAPTER 1

■

CLASSIFICATION OF VOICE DISORDERS

SYMPTOMATOLOGY OF VOICE DISORDERS

Voice change is a common symptom of laryngeal disease. Other symptoms include respiratory distress, cough with variable forms of expectorations, dysphagia, and/or pain related to the larynx. These symptoms are of interest to laryngologists, speech pathologists, phoniatricians, and voice coaches and teachers. Regardless of the discipline, voice specialists are interested in voice change because it may allow the specialist to locate the pathology in the larynx, help and provide the details necessary to reaching a correct diagnosis, and, hence, a best choice of therapy.

Presenting Vocal Symptoms

Common vocal symptoms that a specialist will see are:

1. *Dysphonia* (literally, difficult phonation): This may be broadly defined as a perceptually audible change of a patient's habitual voice, as self-judged or judged by his or her listeners. Dysphonic voice may be also described as a voice that fails to meet a patient's vocal demands, personality, age, size, or gender.
2. *Aphonia:* This reflects an inability to phonate. The patient is capable only of producing a type of whisper.
3. *Phonasthenia:* This may be defined as voice fatigue. It may be referred to as a "dysphonia" that is felt in the neck and throat rather than heard by the patients and their listeners. It may be broadly described by the patient as a status in which voice is not coping with the demands of daily life. The patient may experience:

A. Sense of dryness and/or sourness of the throat.
B. Tenderness in the throat and neck around the larynx.
C. Frequent need to clear the throat (hawking).
D. Sensation of sticky secretions (mucus) in the throat that are difficult to swallow, although swallowing food and drinks is not impaired.
E. Inability to continue "speaking" during vocally stressful situations.
F. Increased effort needed to vocalize.
G. In some cases, change of voice after much or stressful speaking.

4. *Dysodia:* This is defined as a change or failure of some aspects of the singing voice, although the speaking voice is intact.

PATHOPHYSIOLOGICAL MODEL OF DYSPHONIA

To fully appreciate the pathophysiology of voice disorders, it is advisable to understand the structure and function of the vocal organ. Because of restricted space in this book, it is impossible to present more than a cursory summary of the relevant aspects, and readers are referred to other sources of information. For laryngeal joints, Sonesson (1959), von Leden and Moore (1961), and Zenker (1964) are suggested. Glottal divisions are covered by Hirano, Kurita, Kiyokawa, and Sato (1986). Vocal fold structure is detailed by Smith (1957) and Hirano (1975). Structure of the ventricle and ventricular bands can be found in Kotby, Kirchner, Kahane, Bassiony, and El-Samma (1991). Neuroanatomy is covered by Yoshida, Tanaka, Saito, Shimazaki, and Hirano (1992). Laryngeal muscles are detailed by Sonninen (1956) and Hirano (1987). Gross vocal fold movements are discussed in Kotby et al. (1992). Vibratory movements of the vocal folds are examined by Smith (1954), Van den Berg, Zantema, and Doornenbal (1957), Titze (1986), and Titze (1988).

The anatomical correlates of dysphonia may fall in one or more of the following categories:

- Changes in the mass of the vocal fold: Dysphonia may result from an increased mass (polyp, edema, etc.) or reduced mass (atrophy).
- Changes in the stiffness of the mucosa: Dysphonia may result from increased stiffness, as in infiltrative lesions of the mucosa (inflammation), or the deeper structures (cancer). Scarring of the mucosa of the vocal fold may also lead to dysphonia caused by increased stiffness.

- Changes in the degree of vocal fold coaptation: Dysphonia may result from a persistent phonatory gap, as in paralysis of the vocal fold or a mass occupying lesion at the edge of the vocal fold (nodule, polyp, etc.), preventing smooth and precise coaptation of the edges during phonation.

Based on information gained over the past two decades it is clear that the prerequisites of "normal" voice production are:

1. Full range of movement of the vocal folds in vertical and lateral dimensions.
2. Presence of a pliable layered structure with ability to change biomechanical properties of superficial layers of mucosa (epithelium and superficial layer of lamina propria) on the deeper more firm structures (thyroarytenoid muscle) of the vocal fold appropriate to pitch, loudness, and phonatory task.
3. Optimal coaptation of the vocal folds' edges.
4. Optimal phonatory adductory force.
5. Optimal expiratory support to guarantee optimal air flow across the glottis.
6. Optimal timing between the phonatory adduction of the vocal folds and the phonatory exhalation.
7. Optimal tuning of the laryngeal muscles (internal and external) to adjust the vocal fold length, mass, and tension necessary for the intended vocal duties (Kotby, 1986).

It is interesting to note that three (1–3) of the above-mentioned factors are directly related to the "instrument" (vocal folds) with four (4–7) related to the way the "player" (the subject) uses the "instrument." Accordingly, the causes of dysphonia may be organic in nature (due to disturbance in the above prerequisites related to the instrument) or nonorganic (functional) in nature (due to disturbances in the above prerequisites related to the player) (Figure 1–1) or a combination of the two.

ETIOLOGY OF VOICE DISORDERS

An essential prerequisite for selecting the treatment of choice from the available therapeutic armamentarium is having a working outline of the different etiological categories of voice disorders (Figure 1–2). Etiology is divided into three main groups:

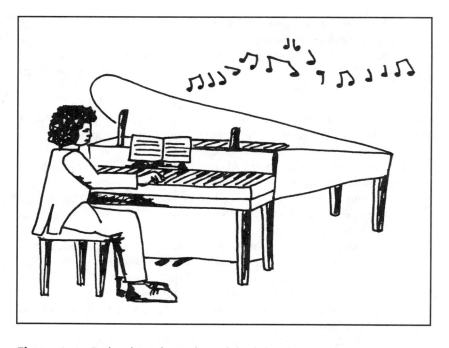

Figure 1–1. Pathophysiological model of dysphonia. The cause of disagreeable tunes may be due to defects in (1) The instrument—organic factors. (2) The player—nonorganic (functional) factors.

1. Organic voice disorders.
2. Nonorganic (functional) voice disorders.
3. Minimal Associated Pathological Lesions (MAPLs).

Organic Voice Disorders

The organic class includes the disorders of voice in which there are detectable morphological changes in the vocal apparatus, usually the vocal folds (Table 1–1).

Two subgroups of organic voice disorders need further clarification, as they frequently emerge as a major indication for the application of the Accent Method (AM) of voice therapy. These are:

1. Neurological disorders of the larynx.
2. Dysplasia of the vocal fold.

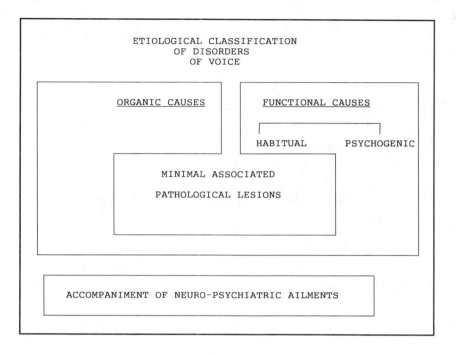

Figure 1–2. An outline of the classification of disorders of voice.

Neurological Disorders of the Larynx

An outline of the categories of neurological ailments that may affect the larynx is given in Tables 1–2 and 1–3.

The motor disorders of the larynx represent the more important clinical category. It includes deficits in mobility, tone, disturbed smoothness, and/or programming of the motor act involving one or both vocal folds. Voice involvement in these cases may be an element of dysarthrophonia (Darley, Aronson, & Brown, 1975). Breakdown of the motor control of the larynx may also be in the form of dystonia. For example, it has been argued that spasmodic dysphonia with its two major types, adductor and abductor, is thought to be a manifestation of laryngeal dystonia (Aronson, 1985).

Symptomatology The symptomatology of impaired motor control of the vocal folds manifests itself either as:

Table 1–1. Organic voice disorders

A. Congenital malformations
  1. Sulcus glottideus
  2. Congenital laryngeal webbing
  3. Cri-du-chat syndrome
  4. Congenital laryngeal cysts and laryngoceles
  5. Congenital laryngeal stridor (Laryngomalacia)

B. Traumatic conditions
  1. Mechanical trauma
     a. Blunt physical trauma
     b. Sharp, cut wounds and stabs
     c. **Vocal trauma** from vocal fold collision against each other.
  2. Physical trauma
     a. Thermal (burns)
     b. Chemical (caustics)
     c. Irradiation

C. Inflammatory Causes
  1. Acute laryngitis
  2. Chronic laryngitis
     a. Specific
     b. Nonspecific

D. Laryngeal allergy

E. Laryngeal tumors
  1. Benign
     a. Papilloma
     b. Others
  2. Dysplasia
  3. Malignant
     a. Carcinoma
     b. Others

F. Neurological disorders of the larynx

G. Endocrinopathies
  1. Thyroid gland dysfunction
  2. Parathyroid gland dysfunction
  3. Pituitary gland dysfunction
  4. Gonadal dysfunction
  5. Virilizing anabolic drugs
  6. Premenstrual changes

H. Status postlaryngectomy

Table 1–2. Etiology of neurological disorders of the larynx

I. Motor Disorders
  A. Upper Motor Neuron Lesions involving:
    • Pyramidal system
    • Extrapyramidal system
    • Cerebellar system
  B. Lower Motor Neuron Lesions involving:
    • Brain stem nuclei
    • Peripheral laryngeal nerves (Table 1–3)
    • Neuromuscular junction
    • Laryngeal muscles

II. Sensory Disorders
  Paraesthesia, hyperthesia, and dysthesia.
  These may be elements of the condition of phonasthenia (vocal fatigue).

Table 1–3. Etiology of recurrent laryngeal nerve palsy

	1 %	2 %	3 %
1. Central	1.2	7.0	8.7
2. Peripheral	98.8	93.0	91.3
Idiopathic	41.3	13.0	4.0
Tumors	17.2	24.5	14.4
Surgery	22.5	20.5	58.2
Trauma	2.30	10.0	9.0
Endotracheal intubation	11.10	—	—
Chest disease	23.0	12.0	1.9
Miscellaneous	—	11.0	3.0

Note. The data in column 1 are from "Recurrent Laryngeal Nerve Paralysis: A 10-year Review of 564 Patients," by M. Yamada, M. Hirano, and H. Ohkubo, 1983. *Auris. Nasus. Larynx* (Tokyo), 10(Suppl.), 1–15.

The data in column 2 are from "The Nervus Vagus," by J. Claes and P. Jaco, 1986, *Acta Oto-rhino-laryngology* (Belgium) *40*, 216.

The data in column 3 are from *E.M.G. of the larynx*, p. 201, by P. H. Dejonckere. Louvain, Belgium: Marc Pietteur.

1. Dys/aphonia, with or without dysphagia and laryngeal over-flow, when the outcome of the disturbed mobility is a persistent glottal waste.
2. Dyspnea and stridor, with variable degrees of strained voice, when the outcome of the disturbed mobility is a persistent glottal stenosis.

The severity of the symptoms in either case may be influenced by several factors:

1. *The laterality of the lesion:* Unilateral lesions give rise to a tremendous range of symptoms. On occasion, these lesions may be discovered on routine examination of the larynx and be asymptomatic. Other lesions, which displace the affected vocal fold to a more lateral position may be completely disabling. Bilateral lesions, on the other hand, may give rise to serious problems, even though voice may be relatively normal.
2. *The degree of the neuropathology:* Symptoms are usually less severe when there is some residual movement compared to when the vocal fold is completely immobile and fixed.
3. *The position of the immobile vocal fold:* The position of the immobile vocal fold is a crucial factor in determining the clinical picture and influences management, including the choice of the Accent Method (AM) over alternative techniques.

If the immobile vocal fold occupies an extremely divergent position in full adduction or full abduction, more severe symptoms may result than the situation when the fold adopts a less extreme position. The position of the vocal fold determines the resultant glottal configuration, with a concomitant effect on dysfunction and symptomatology.

Specific positions have been used to describe the immobile, fixed vocal fold: the paramedian position (1 mm from the midline), the intermedian position (when the vocal fold is fixed between full adduction and full abduction), and the cadaveric position (when the vocal fold is in a flaccid and abducted position) (Howard, 1987). Unfortunately, these positions can rarely, if ever, be observed in clinical practice in such a specific categorical way.

The work of Mukasa and Ueda (1964) helps explain clinical observations. They demonstrated that cadaveric positions of the vocal folds varied and were not in the flaccid abducted posture; the positions varied from midline to full abduction. Such a finding may be explained by anatomical variations in the crico-arytenoid joint and ligaments. In the living, the degree and distribution of a neuropathological lesion may be another factor leading to the diversity of the positions of the paralytic vocal fold. Accordingly, it is suggested that the position of the immobile (paralytic) vocal fold in terms of its distance, in ratio to its length, from the glottic midline posteriorly be used.

Laryngoscopic Image Patients with motor disorders of the larynx may present with some changes in glottal configurations. These changes should be kept in mind when the clinician is applying the Accent Method (AM) for the treatment of motor disorders of the larynx. Changes in gross movements of the vocal folds and configuration of the glottis seen in laryngoscopic examination are described below.

A. *Residual movement of the affected vocal fold:* Variable degrees of residual movement of one or the other of the affected vocal folds may be observed. The side, range, and direction of this movement may influence the choice of the treatment modality and may affect the results of the application of the Accent Method (AM).

B. *Position of the immobile vocal fold:* The immobile (paralytic) vocal fold following recurrent laryngeal nerve affection may adopt any position from paramedian to full abduction depending on the factors mentioned above (Table 1–4). There is a tendency for improved prognosis when the immobile vocal fold adopts a position closer to the glottal midline (Dejonckere, 1987; Wendler, Volprecht, Notzel, Klein, & Fuchs, 1984). Superior laryngeal nerve affection, on the other hand, does not usually give rise to a specific glottal configuration or a particular position (Hirano, Nozoe, Shin, & Maeyama, 1987).

Table 1–4. Relative incidence of the position of the paretic vocal fold

	1 %	2 %
Median	8.5	8.39
Intermediate	15.75	22.58
Paramedian	77.75	60.06
Lateral	—	0.97

Note. Data in column 1 are from "Stimmlippen Lahmungen in der Phoniatrische Praxis," by J. Wendler, I. Vollprecht, M. Notzel, K. Klein, and R. Fuchs, 1984, *Folia Phoniatrica* (Basel), *36*, pp. 74–83.

Data in column 2 are from *E.M.G. of the Larynx* by P. H. Dejonckere, 1987, p. 201. Louvain, Belgium: Marc Pietteur.

C. *Functional glottal configuration:* (1) The size of the maximum available **respiratory glottis**, measured posteriorly in terms of millimeter or ratio measurements, may influence the presenting symptomatology and the plan of intervention. (2) The size of the **phonatory glottal "waste"** or opening relative to the overall size of the vocal folds, may also influence the choice of the treatment modality and the therapeutic results of the Accent Method (AM).

D. *The vertical level of the vocal fold:* The immobile vocal fold may lie at a different vertical plane compared to the unaffected side. The glottal configuration resulting from the combined horizontal and vertical positions of the immobile vocal fold may influence the symptomatology and the choice and results of intervention.

E. *The girth of the vocal fold:* Long-standing lower motor neurone lesions may lead to atrophy of the vocal fold muscles with possible reduction of the fold girth and mass. Any changes in the girth of the vocal fold should be observed and, if possible, measured, as the situation may affect the plan of intervention and the results of therapy utilizing the Accent Method (AM).

F. *Arytenoid movement and position:* In unilateral involvement of the vocal folds, asymmetry of movement and position of the affected "arytenoid mass," relative to the unaffected side may be observed during adductory phonatory movements. The unaffected "arytenoid mass" may move forward and downward, overcrossing the affected one. The latter may adopt an exaggerated forward overhanging position, concealing part of the posterior aspect of the affected vocal fold. The magnitude of these movements and postures may influence the results of therapy.

Stroboscopic Changes   Stroboscopic examination reveals—with greater precision— the size, shape, and place of glottal gaps. A fluttering movement with considerable amplitude of movement instead of the glottal mucosal wave may be seen on the affected side. In unilateral cases, especially with partial neurological lesions, stroboscopy may reveal asymmetry (in amplitude and phase) of glottic vibrations.

The **reappearance** of the glottic wave on the affected side is a good prognostic sign indicating reinnervation with return of tone to the affected muscle (Fex, 1970). Increased tone of the flaccid muscle furnishes the necessary difference in mechanical properties (firm muscle [body], placid mucosa [cover]) needed for the production of glottic mucosal waves. This may reappear 2–3 weeks prior to the observation of gross movement of the vocal fold (Hirano, 1981).

Dysplasia of the Vocal Fold

The Accent Method (AM) can play an important role in alleviating one of the predisposing factors in dysplasia—namely, faulty vocal technique. Consequently, the salient features of this condition are discussed briefly.

Dysplasia is a condition characterized by distorted molding of the layered structure of the stratified squamous epithelium. Several terms have been used to describe this condition such as pachydermia, leukoplakia, acanthosis, and atypia (Figure 1–3). These terms may not be highly descriptive and may raise some misunderstanding; hence the term "dysplasia" is favored in the following description.

Dysplasia, which is an atypical form of hyperplasia, usually results from long-standing laryngeal irritation, such as smoking (Stell & Watt, 1984) and vocal abuse and misuse. The pathological changes seen usually are patchy in distribution, mainly involving the vocal folds. Lehmann, Pidoux, and Widmann (1981) classified dysplasia into three grades of severity. The parameters that are taken into account when grading dysplasia include (Table 1–5):

A. The extent of the changes across the thickness of the epithelium.
B. The degree of nuclear irregularity (dyskariosis, pleomorphism).
C. The degree of active mitotic figures (atypia).
D. The degree of keratosis and parakeratosis.
E. The loss of polarity of the basal layer of the epithelium.

The main presenting symptoms of dysplasia are variable degrees of dysphonia and phonasthenia. Laryngeal examination may reveal whitish, irregular umbilicated small masses, reddish patches, or diffuse swelling of one or both vocal folds. Stroboscopic examination may reveal localized asymmetries of the glottal wave, with occasional independent "rocking" movement of the dysplastic patch.

Nonorganic (Functional) Voice Disorders

This class includes the disorders of voice for which there is no detectable organic pathology in the larynx early in the pathogenesis of the disorders. Later, lesions, such as vocal nodules, may develop. This group represents one of the major indications for the therapeutic application of the Accent Method (AM), thus warranting special attention and description.

Nonorganic (functional) voice disorders as a disease entity has been long recognized (Brodnitz, 1971; Greene, 1980; Fritzell, 1973; Froeschels, 1940). The term "functional dysphonia" is usually applied

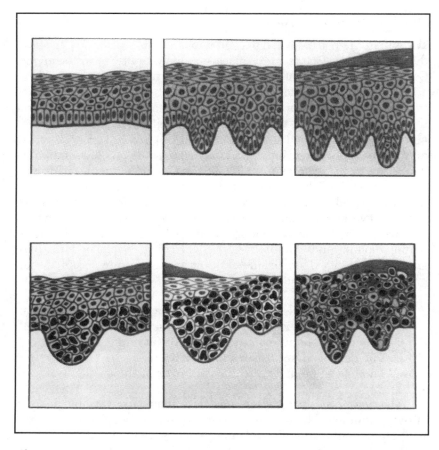

Figure 1–3. Diagram of the histological classification of the grades of dysplasia. *Note.* From *Larynx, Microlaryngoscopy and Histopathology* (p. 43), by W. Lehmann, J. M. Pidoux, and J. J. Widmann, 1981, Cadempino, Switzerland: Inpharzam Medical Publications S. A. Copyright 1981 by Inpharzam Medical Publications S. A. Reprinted with permission.

when a voice complaint is present with no apparent structural change in the larynx. This condition results from the faulty use of a healthy larynx (Murphy, 1964). Moses (1954) suggested that anxiety and neurosis are important factors in the etiology of functional dysphonia. Other predisposing factors are summarized in Table 1–6.

Functional dysphonia, disorder with absence of an organic lesion, has been classified in a variety of different ways. Perello (1962) has used the terms phonoponosis (for voice disorders due to excessive

Table 1–5. Classification of dysplasia

---

(1) Dysplasia grade I (Mild dysplasia)
- Hyperplasia of the malpighian layer reaching up to $^1/_3$ of the thickness of the epithelium (acanthosis)
- Disturbed polarity of basal cells
- Mild hyper- and parakeratosis

(2) Dysplasia grade II (Moderate dysplasia)
- Hyperplasia of the malpighian layer reaching up to $^2/_3$ of the thickness of the epithelium (acanthosis)
- Lost polarity of the basal cells
- Moderate cellular polymorphism (dyskariosis)
- Increased rate of mitosis
- Moderate hyper- and parakeratosis

(3) Dysplasia grade III (Severe dysplasia)
- Hyperplasia of the malpighian layer reaching the surface of the epithelium
- Lost polarity of basal cells
- Stronger cell polymorphism (dyskariosis)
- Higher rates of mitosis (atypia)
- Marked keratosis
- Severely disturbed epithelial architecture
- Grade III is in fluid transition with the so-called carcinoma in situ, which is still a noninvasive condition.

Note. Adapted from "Larynx, microlaryngoscopy and histopathology," by W. Lehmann, J. M. Pidoux, & J. J. Widmann, (1981). Cadempino, Switzerland: Inpharzam Medical Publications.

vocal strain) and phononeurosis (for the psychogenic voice disorders). Luchsinger and Arnold (1965) recognized a habitual and a psychogenic division of functional voice disorders. Fritzell (1973) described five subgroups: hyperfunctional, hypofunctional dysphonia, phonasthenia, hyperfunctional childhood dysphonia, and mutational dysphonia. Damsté and Lerman (1975) identified two functional categories, hyperkinetic and hypokinetic, with several subcategories. Aronson (1985) identified a psychogenic category of voice disorders having a functional background, which was further subdivided into two classes: emotional stress and psychoneurosis. Despite the widespread use of functional voice disorders terminology, its precise definition or even its existence is still doubted by some clinicians.

Table 1–6. Predisposing factors of nonorganic (functional) voice disorders (Protocol for Voice Evaluation; Appendix 1)

1. **Vocal abuse behaviors**
   a. Screaming: conscious and unconscious
   b. Throat clearing

2. **Vocal misuse (faulty) behaviors**
   a. Faulty respiration
      i. Speaking on low lung volumes
      ii. Tense upper-chest breathing
   b. Faulty loudness
      i. Excessively soft (personality related)
      ii. Excessively loud (Personality/environment related)
   c. Faulty pitch
      i. Excessively low pitch
      ii. Excessively high pitch
      iii. Mutational disorders
   d. Faulty phonatory mode
      i. Hard glottal attack
      ii. Vocal fry usually at the end of the utterance

3. **Smoking (active or passive)**

4. **Environmental pollution:**
   • Physical: noise (Lombard effect)
   • Climatic: dryness and cold air
   • Chemical: dusts and fumes

5. **Psychological emotional stress and personality traits:**
   • Occupational stress.
   • Generalized or specific anxiety
   • Personal stresses

6. **Biological factors:**
   • Gastroeosophageal reflux
   • Allergy
   • Rheumatoid arthritis
   • Alcohol and diet
   • Autonomic nervous dysfunction affecting laryngeal secretions and vascularity

I (Kotby, 1986) have classified nonorganic (functional) voice disorders into: **habitual voice disorders**, which are further subdivided into:

1. Hyperfunctional childhood dysphonia.
2. Mutational voice disorders.

3. Hyperfunctional dysphonia.
4. Hypofunctional dysphonia.
5. Phonasthenia.
6. Ventricular dysphonia.
7. Habitual aphonia.

and **psychogenic voice disorders,** which may be described under:

1. Psychogenic dysphonia.
2. Psychogenic aphonia.

Habitual Nonorganic (Functional) Voice Disorders

Hyperfunctional Childhood Dysphonia This condition is typically seen in children who are gregarious and who are misusing and/or abusing their voices and is evidenced equally in both sexes (Kotby, El-Sady, Abd El-Rahman, Abd El-Nasser, & Dawod, 1994). The condition affects the speaking as well as the singing voice (Wilson, 1987). The child with hyperfunctional dysphonia has, however, no subjective complaint. The child is referred to a clinician by a teacher or parents because of a "hoarse voice." Auditory perceptual assessment (APA) reveals strained, leaky voice, which may be also irregular (rough) with an apparent low frequency. The vocal folds may show broad-based nodules at the middle of the free edge, with incomplete glottal closure caused by these nodules. Some cases may only show increased vascular markings and slight diffuse swelling of the vocal fold mucosa. Once the swellings have developed, the voice is perceived to be lower in pitch and loudness. The psychoacoustic measures of frequency show the voice frequently falls within normal limits. The acoustic amplitude and frequency perturbation show significant increase compared to normal voices (Saleh, 1991). Before detemining an actual diagnosis of this condition, it is important to exclude other organic lesions (web, sulcus, cyst) as a cause for the dysphonia in these children (Fritzell, 1973).

Treatment for these children is controversial. One school of thought holds that clinicians should adopt a "wait and see" stance as many children grow out of this disorder. The other school of thought contends that only boys outgrow nodules, and poor voice has an adverse effect on self-concept development and limits career choices. When treatment is recommended, it includes reassurance, counseling, follow-up, and direct symptom management. Voice therapy may be particularly well advised for children who are interested in singing and who have enough motivation to undergo therapy.

For children, endolaryngeal microsurgical removal of a nodule is rarely needed. When this line of treatment is justified, it is usually for older youth (11–12 years) who have been unresponsive to traditional treatment and who have relatively fibrotic (whitish) large and asymmetrical nodules. The child should be persuaded to follow proper voice hygiene and voice therapy after surgery.

Mutational Voice Disorders   Mutational voice disorders are found mainly in adolescent males. Some factors such as psychological, endocrine disorders, learning problems, and hearing loss are thought to share in causation (Aronson, 1985).

It should be pointed out that the majority of those young men are perfectly healthy. A patient will complain of a weak, unclear voice. Rarely, a patient will complain of a high-pitched, girlish character of voice. Auditory perceptual assessment by the clinician reveals a high-pitched voice with or without register breaks.

Laryngeal examination reveals normal vocal folds with smooth edge. There is usually a diffuse, pinkish discoloration of the vocal fold mucosa caused by a high degree of laryngeal tension used to produce the abnormally high voice. The larynx usually is felt elevated in the neck. Amplitude perturbation measures show significant rise in mutational voice disorders (Saleh, 1991).

Management is usually in the form of reassurance and counseling together with voice therapy. The elevated larynx may be guided to its expected lower position by gentle digital manipulation. This may help the patient to find his habitual chest voice, which can then be stabilized by behavior readjustment voice therapy.

Hyperfunctional Dysphonia   Brodnitz (1971) did not identify hyperfunction as a diagnosis in itself, but a term that describes a complex vocal symptom. Despite his precaution, this condition is usually clinically identifiable as an independent category. It is more commonly seen in males than females in the fourth and fifth decades of life. Vocal abuse and misuse; noisy, dry, and dusty environment; and stressful speaking situations are factors that may predispose to vocal hyperfunction (Moses, 1954). The usual complaint is dysphonia and phonasthenic manifestations. The voice is characterized by being strained and leaky with tendency to hard glottal attacks (Prater & Swift, 1987). It may also be low-pitched with tendency to increased loudness.

The vocal folds may look and behave normally. There may be increased vascular markings of the lining mucosa and phonatory hyperadduction of the vocal folds with a tendency of ventricular bands aproximation. Subtle stroboscopic deviations in the form of asymmetry of the glottal wave may be seen. Acoustically, there are significant changes in the amplitude and frequency perturbation measures (Saleh, 1991). Management is usually in the form of behavior readjustment voice therapy.

Hypofunctional Dysphonia This condition is seen more frequently in patients in the third decade of life. It has been claimed that the condition results from long-standing hyperfunctional dysphonia, which may lead to muscle fatigue and inadequate muscular control of the glottis during phonation. This may produce a persistent phonatory gap and a short closed phase in the phonatory vibratory cycle (Fritzell, 1973).

A patient will complain of a weak voice with accompanied symptoms of voice fatigue (phonasthenia). Auditory perceptual assessment by the clinician reveals a breathy voice with reduced intensity. Laryngoscopic examination reveals incomplete glottal closure during phonation. Stroboscopic examination may show reduced vibratory amplitude. Management is essentially by behavior readjustment voice therapy.

Phonasthenia In its isolated form, this condition is a relatively common voice problem. Although no demographic data exist, it is thought to be equally present in both sexes. Long-standing vocal abuse, misuse, smoking, and exposure to environmental pollution are common predisposing factors. Vocal fatigue symptoms (phonasthenia) may present as a primary complaint or may accompany several nonorganic, organic, and MAPLs conditions. Some of the phonasthenic symptoms described below may also result from psychological stress and anxiety. The symptoms of vocal fatigue (phonasthenic manifestations) are in the form of:

1. Voice fatigue following prolonged voice use: The patient feels exhausted and wants to stop talking. The patient may also note voice cracks and reduced vocal range.
2. Dryness, tightness, and soreness in the throat.
3. Frequent throat clearing.
4. Feeling of persistent sticky mucus in the throat. Despite the difficulty in swallowing this sticky mucus, swallowing fluids or solids is free (Brodnitz, 1971; Kotby, 1986).

Voice is generally normal, but it may be strained or breathy. Laryngoscopic examination is essentially normal, but may reveal increased vascular markings of the mucosa. Subtle stroboscopic deviations in the form of asymmetries of the glottal mucosal wave may be observed. Acoustic studies show a significant rise in the measure of fractal dimension (Saleh, 1991).

Management is in the form of reassurance and behavior readjustment voice therapy. In anxious and neurotic patients, minor tranquilizers may be resorted to as an adjuvant treatment.

Ventricular Dysphonia (dysphonia plica ventricularis)   This condition is known also as false fold phonation (Boone, 1988, McFarlane, 1988). It occurs as:

1. A manifestation of prolonged hyperfunctional voice disorder.
2. A compensation for nonvibrating vocal folds as in:
   a. Vocal fold paralysis or large glottal gap from other causes.
   b. Removal of the vocal fold (cordectomy).
   c. Postirradiation reaction and fibrosis.

It occurs more commonly in males. The main symptom is deep "hoarse" voice with or without symptoms of vocal fatigue. APA reveals strained, leaky, rough, and low-pitched voice. Diplophonia may be observed. The laryngoscopic findings point to phonatory tightness with hyperadduction of the glottis and supraglottal structures. Phonatory contact and vibration of the ventricular bands may be observed. This may be due to hyperadduction or actual hypertrophy of the ventricular bands.

Management is basically behavior readjustment voice therapy. In a case of true excessive ventricular band hypertrophy, adequate surgical reduction via direct microlaryngoscopy may be resorted to.

Functional Habitual Aphonia (FHA)   FHA is a temporary loss of phonation independent of an organic laryngeal pathology (Kaiser, Kotby, & Kotby, 1978). It is significantly found more frequently in females. Most of the cases are of habitual nature. The presence and severity of underlying psychiatric ailments is difficult to discern. Acute laryngitis, acute vocal abuse (trauma), postoperative status (as after extensive extirpation of the vocal fold mucosa), and sudden psychogenic stress are common predisposing factors. The temporary aphonia caused by these factors may continue after the etiological basis has long disappeared. The patients continue to be aphonic because of lack of secondary gains of impaired voice or because of lack of appropriate proprioceptive feedback from vocal fold contact during the aphonia. This lack of proprioceptive feedback perpetuates the condition (Boone, 1988). Greene (1980) believes that the greatest incidence of FHA is between the ages of 18–34 years, while Kaiser, Kotby, & Kotby (1978) found that the greatest incidence is between 12–18 years. The FHA patient is capable only of producing a whisper, which may be hyper- or hypofunctional. The nonverbal phonatory activities of the larynx such as coughing, laughing, and crying are characteristically intact.

Laryngoscopic examination reveals normal vocal folds. There is usually phonatory waste of various degrees; the vocal folds fail to approximate during the aborted phonatory attempts. The glottal chink may be in one of a variety of positions and is not necessarily restricted to the typical whisper configuration. However, complete glottal closure occurs during coughing or gagging.

Management of functional habitual aphonia is achieved by several methods. Digital side pressure on the larynx (to enhance glottal contact), and bilateral masking of the ears (to abolish self-monitoring) may prove successful. In some cases, voice can be reinstated by starting from a very high-pitched falsetto that helps the patient to feel vocal fold contact with reassurance via the proprioceptive feedback. The patient is then guided to produce a suitable chest register. Vocal fold contact can be also achieved by other techniques, such as humming or repetitive short nonphonatory glottal attacks. It is recommended, though not essential, to attempt voice restoration at the first session of therapy (Boone, 1988; Brondnitz, 1971; Greene, 1980). Behavior readjustment voice therapy may be used to stabilize the regained voice.

Psychogenic (Nonorganic) Voice Disorders

Psychogenic Dysphonia   The voice clinician may encounter a patient presenting with a bizarre vocal behavior although the larynx looks normal under examination. Noncommunicative vocal activities such as coughing and laughing are free. This type of voice problem does not allow classification under any of the aforementioned categories of nonorganic (functional) dysphonia. The condition, which is more common in females, is usually of sudden onset (Schalén & Andersson, 1992). Following proper assessment to exclude other etiological factors the management comprises proper counseling and reassurance. Attempting to guide the patient to find his or her natural physiological habitual voice production by establishing good phonatory contact may help in restoring voice. For these cases, stabilization of the regained voice by behavior readjustment voice therapy, such as the Accent Method (AM), may be needed.

Psychogenic Aphonia   Nonorganic aphonia may be a presentation of a specific psychiatric ailment (conversion hysteria). This type of aphonia is rather persistent and its management usually requires cooperation between the voice clinician and the psychiatrist.

Voice Disorders Accompanying Psychiatric Diseases   Some psychiatric diseases that affect personality and mood (e.g., depression, catatonia) may cause a change of voice. In these conditions, the care of the voice problem, which is of secondary importance, should be attempted after the management of the primary psychiatric disease.

Minimal Associated Pathological Lesions (MAPLs)

Long-standing, nonorganic (functional) voice disorders may lead to the creation of detectable organic changes. These lesions are usually associated with and might have been predisposed by long-standing nonorganic vocal dysfunction. These lesions are benign and are usually of a limited extent. From the morphological and pathogenic points of view, this group occupies a position somewhere between the organic and nonorganic (functional) groups.

Vocal nodules, polyps, contact granuloma, Reinke's edema, and vocal fold cysts are examples of these lesions (Kotby, Ghaly, & Barakah, 1980; Mossallam, Kotby, Ghaly, Nassar, & Barakah, 1986) (Table 1–7). These lesions are grouped together because they share certain common features:

Table 1–7: Minimal Associated Pathological Lesions (MAPLs)

1.	Vocal fold polyp
2.	Vocal fold nodules a. Juvenile type b. Adult type
3.	Reinke's edema
4.	Contact granuloma (Intubation granuloma!)
5.	Vocal fold cysts
6.	Ventricular dysphonia (!)

1. They have common predisposing factors. Vocal abuse and misuse (vocal trauma) are considered to be the prime factors in the causation of these lesions. Smoking and other laryngeal irritants may also play a role (Kleinsasser, 1991; Kotby, Ghali & Barakah, 1980; Prater & Swift, 1987), although the exact nature of this role is not yet understood.

2. They have related histopathological features. These lesions were previously classified as benign tumors of the vocal fold (Holinger & Johnston, 1951; Stewart, 1957) and as a manifestation of chronic, nonspecific inflammation of the larynx (Ellis, 1952; Salmon, 1979). There is accumulated evidence, however, that such lesions are of a nonneoplastic, noninflammatory nature (Kleinsasser, 1991; Kotby, Nassar, Seif, Helal, & Saleh, 1988; Mossallam, Kotby, Ghaly, Nassar, & Barakah, 1986).

3. They have similar presenting symptoms (dysphonia with or without phonasthenia).

4. They usually require similar lines of treatment and management, namely a combination of minor surgical intervention and behavior readjustment voice therapy.

5. They share a common favorable prognosis.

Accordingly, MAPLs is used to group these lesions that share several common features. The terminology reflects two major features:

A. The pathological changes are usually minimal or at least benign in nature.

B. These lesions are caused by or are in association with long-standing faulty vocal habits.

REFERENCES

Aronson, A. E. (1985). *Clinical voice disorders: An inter-disciplinary approach* (2nd ed.). New York: Thieme-Stratton, Inc.

Boone, D. R. (1988). *The voice and voice therapy* (4th ed.). Englewood Cliffs, NJ: Prentice-Hall.

Brodnitz, F. S. (1971). *Vocal rehabilitation* (4th ed.). Rochester, MN: American Academy of Ophthalmology and Otolaryngology.

Claes, J., & Jaco, P. (1986). The nervus vagus. *Acta Oto-rhino-laryngologica*, Belgium, *40*, 216.

Damsté, P. H., & Lerman, J. W. (1975). *An introduction to voice pathology.* Springfield, IL: Charles C. Thomas.

Darley, F. L., Aronson, A. E., & Brown, J. R. (1975). *Motor speech disorders.* Philadelphia: W. B. Saunders.

Dejonckere, P. H. (1987). *E.M.G. of the larynx* (p. 201). Louvain, Belgium: Marc Pietteur.

Ellis, M. (1952). Chronic non-specific laryngitis. In W. G. Scott Brown (Ed.), *Scott Brown's diseases of the ear, nose and throat* (Vol. 1) (pp. 590–618). London: Butterworth.

Fex, S. (1970). Judging the movements of vocal cords in larynx paralysis. *Acta Oto-laryngologica* (Stockholm), (Suppl. 263), 82.

Fritzell, B. (1973). *Foniatri for medicinare*. Stockholm: Amqvist & Wiksell.

Froeschels, E. (1940). Laws in the appearance and the development of voice hyperfunctions. *Journal of Speech Disorders, 1*.

Greene, M. C. L. (1980). *The voice and its disorders* (4th ed.). Philadelphia: J.B. Lippincott Company.

Hirano, M. (1975). Phonosurgery, basic and clinical investigations. *Otologia Fukuoka,* (Suppl. 1), (pp. 239–242).

Hirano, M. (1981). *Clinical examination of voice*. New York: Springer-Verlag.

Hirano, M. (1987). The laryngeal muscle in singing. In M. Hirano, J. A. Kirchner, & D. M. Bless (Eds.), *Neurolaryngology: Recent advances* (p. 209). Boston: Little, Brown and Company.

Hirano, M., Kurita, S., Kiyokawa, K., & Sato, K. (1986). Posterior glottis: Morphological study in excised human larynges. *Annals of Otology, Rhinology & Laryngology, 95,* 576.

Hirano, M., Nozoe, I., Shin, T., & Maeyama, T. (1987). Electromyography for laryngeal paralysis. In M. Hirano, J. A. Kirchner, & D. M. Bless (Eds.), *Neurolaryngology: Recent advances* (p. 232). Boston: Little, Brown and Company.

Holinger, P. H., & Johnston, K. C. (1951). Benign tumors of the larynx. *Annals of Otology, Rhinology & Laryngology, 60,* 496.

Howard, D. (1987). Neurological affections of the pharynx and larynx. In J. Ballantyne & J. Groves (Eds.), *Scott Brown's diseases of the ear, nose, and throat* (4th ed.) (p. 529). London: Butterworth.

Kaiser, W., Kotby, M. N., & Kotby, I. (1978). Functional aphonia. Diagnostic and therapeutic considerations. *Proceedings of the Second Annual Ain Shams Medical Congress* (Vol. II) (p. 21).

Kleinsasser, O. (1991). Restoration of the voice in benign lesions of the vocal folds by endolaryngeal microsurgery. *Journal of Voice, 5*(3), 257.

Kotby, M. N. (1986). Voice disorders: Recent diagnostic advances. *Egyptian Journal of Otolaryngology, 3*(1), 69.

Kotby, M. N, Barakah, M. A., Abou El-Ella, M. Y., Khidr A. A., & Hegazi M. A. (1990). Aerodynamic analysis of voice disorders. In T. Sacristàn, J. J. Alvarez-Vicent, J. Bartual, F. Antoli-Candela, & L. Rubio (Eds.), Otorhino-laryngology, Head and Neck Surgery. *Proceedings of XIV World Congress of Otorhinolaryngology, Head and Neck Surgery* (Vol II) (pp. 20–41). Amsterdam: Kugler and Ghedini Publication.

Kotby, M. N., Bassiouny, S. E., Amin, M., Garrett, D., Kirchner, J. A., & Kahane, J. C. (1992). Pattern of gross displacement of the vocal fold in adduction and abduction movements. *Acta Otolaryngologica* (Stockholm), *112,* 349.

Kotby, M. N., El-Sady, S. R., Abd El-Rahman, A. G., Abd El-Nasser, H., Dawood, A. A., & Helal, E. H. (1994). Pediatric vocal fold nodules: Diagnostic profile and alternative lines of management. In Jacob Sadé (Ed.), *Infections in childhood ear nose and throat aspects* (pp. 354–361). Amsterdam, The Netherlands: Elsevier Science B.V.

Kotby, M. N., Ghali, A. F., & Barakah, M. (1980). Re-categorization of non-malignant organic vocal fold changes in dysphonia. *The Proceedings of the 18th Congress of International Association of Logopedics and Phoniatrics, Washington, 1*, 525.

Kotby, M. N., Kirchner, J. A., Kahane, J. C., Bassiouny, S. E., & El-Samaa, M. (1991). Histo-anatomical structure of the human laryngeal ventricle. *Acta Otolaryngologica* (Stockholm), *111*, 396.

Kotby, M. N., Nassar, M. A., Seif, E. I., Helal, E. H., & Saleh, M. M. (1988). Ultrastructural features of vocal fold nodules and polyps. *Acta Otolaryngologica (Stockholm), 105*, 477.

Kotby, M. N., Titze, I. R., Abou Rass, Y. A., Saleh M. M., Abd El-Nasser, N. H., & Hegazi M. A. (1991, August). *Diagnostic profile of functional voice disorders*. Paper presented in Collegium Medicorum Theatri (COMET) meeting in Vadstena, Sweden.

Lehmann, W., Pidoux, J. M., & Widmann, J. J. (1981). *Larynx, microlaryngoscopy and histopathology*. Cadempino, Switzerland: Inpharzam Medical Publications.

Luchsinger, R., & Arnold, G. E. (1965). *Voice-speech-language*. Belmont, CA: Wadsworth Publishing Co. Inc.

McFarlane, S. C. (1988). Treatment of benign laryngeal disorders with traditional methods and techniques of voice therapy. *Ear, Nose & Throat Journal, 67*, 425.

Moses, P. J. (1954). *The voice of neurosis*. New York: Grune & Stratton.

Mossallam, I., Kotby, M. N., Ghaly, A. F., Nassar, A. M., & Barakah, M. A. (1986). Histopathological aspects of benign vocal fold lesions associated with dysphonia. In J. A. Kirchner (Ed.), *Vocal fold histopathology* (p. 65). San Diego: College-Hill Press.

Mukasa, T., & Ueda, T. (1964). The position of the vocal cords in cadaver and so-called cadaveric position of the vocal cords. *Journal of Otolaryngology, Japan, 65*, 184.

Murphy, A. T. (1964). *Functional voice disorders*. Englewood Cliffs, NJ: Prentice-Hall.

Perello, J. (1962). Disphonies fonctionelles. *Folia Phoniatrica (Basel), 14*, 150.

Prater, R. J., & Swift, R. W. (1987). *Manual of voice therapy*, (3rd ed.). Boston: Little, Brown & Company.

Saleh, M. S. (1991). *Acoustic analysis of voice in certain types of dysphonia*. Unpublished doctoral dissertation, Faculty of Medicine, Ain Shams University, Cairo.

Salmon, L. F. W. (1979). Chronic laryngitis. In J. Ballantyne & J. Groves (Eds.), *Scott Brown's diseases of the ear, nose and throat* (4th ed.) (Vol. 4) (p. 381). London: Butterworth.

Schalén, L., & Andersson, K. (1992). Differential diagnosis and treatment of psychogenic voice disorder. *Clinical Otolaryngology*, *17*, 225.

Smith, S. (1954). Remarks on the physiology of the vibration of the vocal fold. *Folia Phoniatrica* (Basel), *6*, 166.

Smith, S. (1957). Chest register versus head-register in the membrane-cushion model of the vocal cords. *Folia Phoniatrica* (Basel), *9*, 32.

Sonesson, B. (1959). Die funktionelle anatomie des crico-arytenoid gelenkes. *Zeitschrift Anatomie Entwicklungsgesch*, *121*, 292.

Sonninen, A. A. (1956). The role of the external laryngeal muscle in length adjustment of the vocal cord in singing. *Acta Otolaryngologica* (Stockholm), (Suppl. 130).

Stell, P. M., & Watt, J. (1984). Squamous metaplasia of the subglottic spaces and its relation to smoking. *Annals of Otology, Rhinology & Laryngology*, *93*, 124.

Stewart, J. P. (1957). The histopathology of benign tumors of the larynx. *Journal of Laryngology & Otology*, *17*, 718.

Titze, I. R. (1986). Mean intraglottic pressure in vocal fold oscillation. *Journal of Phonetics*, *14*, 356.

Titze, I. R. (1988). The physics of small amplitude oscillation of the vocal folds. *Journal of the Acoustical Society of America*, *83*(4), 1536.

Van den Berg, J. W., Zantema, J. T., & Doornenbal, F., Jr. (1957). On the air resistance and the Bernoulli effect of the human larynx. *Journal of the Acoustical Society of America*, *29*, 626.

von Leden, H., & Moore, P. (1961). The mechanics of the cricoarytenoid joint. *Archives of Otolaryngology*, *73*, 541.

Wendler, J., Vollprecht, I., Notzel, M., Klein, K., & Fuchs, R. (1984). Stimmlippen lahmungen in der phoniatrische Praxis. *Folia Phoniatrica* (Basel), *36*, 74.

Wilson, D. K. (1987). *Voice problems of children* (3rd ed.) Baltimore: Williams & Wilkins.

Yamada, M., Hirano, M., & Ohkubo, H. (1983). Recurrent laryngeal nerve paralysis. A 10-year review of 564 patients. *Auris. Nasus. Larynx* (Tokyo), 10 (Suppl.), 1–15.

Yoshida, Y., Tanaka, Y., Saito, T., Shimazaki, T.,& Hirano, M. (1992). Peripheral nervous system in the larynx: An anatomical study of the motor, sensory and autonomic nerve fibers. *Folia Phoniatrica* (Basel), *44*(5), 194.

Zenker, W. (1964). Vocal muscle fibers and their motor end plates. In D. W. Brewer (Ed.), *Research potentials in voice physiology* (p. 7). New York: University Press of New York.

CHAPTER 2

■

MANAGEMENT OF VOICE DISORDERS

DIAGNOSIS

In clinical practice, proper diagnosis (assessment) is considered the basis for optimal treatment (intervention), with voice disorders included. During the last few decades, considerable progress has been made in the development of assessment procedures for detecting and describing voice disorders, striving to proceed from subjectivity to objectivity.

The goal of the voice assessment is by no means restricted to a search for an etiological label to the pathology (disease process); assessment encompasses other goals important to describing the degree and severity of the problem and in determining a treatment plan and prognosis. A general review of the goals of the diagnostic procedure of disorders of voice is:

1. Categorizing etiology of the voice ailment and the type of the vocal pathology.
2. Assessing the degree of the functional deficit (degree of the vocal pathology).
3. Choosing of the type and sequence of an intervention program.
4. Monitoring the results of intervention.
5. Drawing adequate prognostic predictions.
6. Understanding the nature of the vocal pathology (research) (Kotby, 1986).

With these goals in mind, one can appreciate the complexity of the diagnostic procedure of voice disorders described in the assessment protocol and accept its evolving nature (See Appendix 1: Protocol for Voice Evaluation).

The assessment protocol is designed to encompass three stages of evaluation of escalating complexity. The diagnostic procedure in each stage briefly follows.

Elementary Diagnostic Procedures

This stage needs no sophisticated equipment. A good deal of relevant information can be collected by noninstrumental measures, provided a clear systematic methodology is applied by a knowledgeable voice clinician. The procedures carried out in this stage of the protocol should be easy to apply in most clinics giving primary voice health care.

Clinical Diagnostic Aids

This stage of the protocol aims at supporting or excluding the diagnostic decision reached at the end of "stage 1." This stage requires some advanced hardware. The procedures carried out at this stage, though usually noninvasive and relatively inexpensive, are recommended to be reserved for specialized voice clinics.

Additional Instrumental Diagnostic Measures

This stage is an option for highly specialized voice laboratories. Though most of the tests are noninvasive, their value as diagnostic tools in routine clinical practice is not yet substantiated. These tools, however, still can fulfill some of the goals of the diagnostic procedure.

TREATMENT OF VOICE DISORDERS

The goal of treating a voice disorder is at least twofold. One should aim at:

A. "Fixing" the vocal organ (instrument), restoring its structural integrity.
B. Reeducating the subject (player), readjusting a faulty vocal behavior.

There are five main avenues to achieve these goals: phonosurgery, pharmacotherapy, supportive technical devices, behavior readjustment voice therapy, and counseling.

PHONOSURGERY

Definition

Phonosurgery refers to the surgical techniques that aim primarily at the improvement of voice or pseudo voice (Isshiki, 1980; Saito, 1977; von Leden, Yanagihara, & Wernre-Kukuk, 1967). The goal of the phonosurgical procedures is to restore the integrity of the vocal organ by:

1. Achieving a smooth edge of the vocal fold with a mobile mucosa and an optimal coaptation of the glottis.
2. Abolishing phonatory glottal gap (waste), or glottal sphincteric incompetence.
3. Restoring a functional respiratory glottis while preserving vocal function.

This section is not a "how to do phonosurgery," rather it is a brief summary of the types of procedures available and the specific goals in making the laryngeal anatomy functional.

Phonosurgical procedures can include the following detailed categories.

Extirpation Endolaryngeal Microphonosurgery

These procedures aim at the removal of small swellings (such as polyps, nodules, or cysts) and aspiration of Reinke's edema to achieve a smooth vocal fold edge with an intact and freely mobile mucosa. Such an intervention also restores the vocal fold mass to its normal limits (Kleinsasser, 1968, 1991).

It should be stressed that the extent of the extirpation (removal) in these procedures has to be minimal both in depth and in surface extension. Deep excisions involving the vocal ligament will heal with a scar that might interfere with the free mobility of the vocal fold mucosa and, hence, the vibratory glottic wave. Such an outcome presents a challenge to the voice clinician by limiting the possibility of optimal postoperative vocal results (Hirano, 1975).

For smoother and quicker healing that promotes better vocal results, with or without postoperative voice therapy, the treatment team should guard against rough handling of the vocal fold mucosa or having a surgical wound with mucosal tags (Bouchayer & Cornut, 1992; Ford & Bless, 1991). Similarly, excessive carbonization should be avoided after laser surgery (Steiner, Jaumann, & Pesch, 1980).

Vocal Fold Augmentation

These procedures aim at reducing small phonatory glottal waste (gap) and correcting localized defects (irregularities) of the vocal fold edge by injecting a variety of inert materials (Arnold, 1962; Brünings, 1911; Ford & Bless, 1986; Fukuda, 1970; Hill, Mayers, & Harris, 1991; Schramm, May, & Lavorato, 1978)

Vocal Fold Debulking and Arytenoidectomy

These procedures aim at the improvement of the laryngeal airway in cases of paralytic persistent glottal stenosis. They aim at widening the posterior glottis, with least disturbance to the anterior phonatory glottis, thus limiting compromise of the postoperative voice results (Kleinsasser, 1968; Motta, 1984; Ossaff, Karlan, & Sisson, 1983).

Vocal Fold Repositioning

This includes a variety of procedures, each with a particular aim in achieving a specific repositioning.

Medial Repositioning of the Vocal Fold (Mediopexy)   This procedure is aimed at correcting big phonatory glottal wastes (gaps). This is an alternative to the procedures discussed under augmentation of the vocal fold. This may be achieved by thyroplasty type I (Isshiki, 1980) or arytenoid adduction (Isshiki, Tanabe, & Sawada, 1978).

Lateral Repositioning of the Vocal Fold (Lateropexy)   This surgery seeks to improve the laryngeal airway in cases of persistent glottal narrowing. This can be achieved by lateral rotation of the arytenoid cartilage (King, 1939) or lateral slinging of the vocal fold (Enjell, 1984).

Neurophonosurgery

This, too, includes a variety of procedures with particular aims.

Remobilization   A paralyzed vocal fold can be reinnervated through a variety of procedures (Attaly et al., 1990; Sato & Ogura, 1978; Tucker, 1977).

Reduction   Hyperadductory movements of the vocal folds in adductory spasmodic dysphonia (SD) can be reduced by several means.

Nerve resection of the trunk of the recurrent laryngeal nerve (RLN) (Dedo, 1976) is one method. Or, there can be resection of a branch of the RLN that innervates an adductor muscle, such as the thyroarytenoid (TA), to reduce the postoperative morbidity following the former procedure (Iwamura, 1986; Iwamura, Takeutchi, Hosoya, Tateoka, & Fukayama, 1986; Takayama, Fukuda, Koawa, & Saito, 1988).

Immobilization of the vocal fold can be accomplished by producing temporary paralysis of the TA muscle through the injection of Botulinum A toxin in that muscle (Blitzer & Brin, 1991; Ford, Bless, & Lowery, 1991; Miller, Woodson, & Jankovic, 1987).

Reconstruction of the Glottis After Partial Laryngectomy

These procedures aim at creating a fixed mass at the side of the laryngectomy, against which the unaffected vibrating vocal fold can meet and coapt properly (Burgess & Yim, 1988; Hirano, 1976).

Postlaryngectomy "Phonosurgery"

These procedures aim at increasing the air flow at the pharyngo-esophageal segment and hence improvement of esophageal "voice" fluency. This can be achieved by creating a tracheoesophageal shunt and the insertion of a prosthesis (Hilgers & Schouwenburg, 1990; Singer, 1983; Singer & Blom, 1980).

Surgical Voice Teamwork

For the optimal practice of phonosurgery, a voice clinician is usually teamed with a phonosurgeon. The team works with the patient in making the choice of the type and extent of the surgical correction needed to optimize the vocal results following phonosurgery. Variable courses of postoperative behavior readjustment voice therapy may also be recommended to augment the surgery.

PHARMACOTHERAPY

Although an important sector of voice disorders is nonorganic, several pharmacological agents have been widely used for the treatment of these ailments. The prescription of these medicines is often based on subjective clinical experience only. There is, nevertheless, a place for pharmacotherapy for the treatment of disorders of voice, if used judiciously. Over the centuries, many popular beliefs have accumulated about the use of certain drinks and simple decoctions for the treatment of voice disorders. Part of the beneficial effects of these drinks is due to their effect on relieving the subjective symptoms of voice fatigue (phonasthenia), especially throat dryness and soreness. Perhaps these drinks work to relieve such symptoms through the simple hydration effect of intake of fluids. Hydration leads to the production of watery (less viscous) secretions in the larynx and the pharynx. Such watery secretions are more easily expelled and relieve the subjective feeling of sticky mucus (veiling) the voice. In this respect, the simple advice of increased fluid intake (overhydration) has stood the test of time as an effective tool to reduce phonasthenic symptoms (Van Lawrence, 1987).

Inhalation therapy is one of the common pharmacotherapy tools. Despite its wide use for several decades, little objective evaluation of its effect and mechanism of action has been published (Brodnitz, 1971). Inhalation therapy may be simple steam inhalation (hot or cold) or medicated steam. The empirical use of tincture benzoine compositum and tincture iodine has no substantiated added beneficial effect. It is claimed that the use of hydrocortisone 2% with a weak vasoconstrictor has good effects on reducing mild laryngeal inflammatory edema. This medicament can be used as a laryngeal inhalant or even as a spray. It should be pointed out, however, that the latter tool is limited to very restricted indications.

Harris (1992) comprehensively reviews the various classes of medicaments that may be used in the treatment of voice disorders. These medicines can fall into the following classes:

1. Agents to liquify mucus to aid ease of expectoration.
2. Cough depressants to control nonproductive, intractable cough, thus reducing an important source of vocal fold trauma.
3. Antiallergic agents to control **evident** allergic manifestations.
4. Antacids and H_2 blockers to control the effects of gastroesophageal reflux.
5. Hormone replacement therapy, especially thyroid and gonadal hormones.
6. Systemic steroid therapy to reduce vocal fold mucosal edema in some selected cases. The rationale and results of treatment await further substantiation.
7. Psychopharmacological agents to alleviate possible concurrent anxiety in selected cases of nonorganic (functional) voice disorders, including phonasthenia.
8. Medicaments for the specific control of some neurological disorders, such as antiparkinsonian agents and agents for the treatment of myasthenia gravis.

In his review, Harris (1992) refers to the unjustified use of antibiotics in the treatment of voice disorders. It is equally important to point out that the indiscriminate use of salicylates may produce some side effects (submucosal bleeding) that may cause dysphonia rather than relieving it (Brodnitz, 1971).

TECHNICAL AID DEVICES

In the management of voice disorders, some technical devices may be used for complete vocal rehabilitation. Electronic and mechanical vibrators can be used as serviceable and feasible alternatives for "sound" production after total laryngectomy. The mechanical vibrator (Tokyo larynx) offers a specially handy and inexpensive tool (Blom, 1978; Broman, Kotby, & Arlin, 1977).

The use of a portable sound amplification system might be recommended for some patients with excessive vocal demands, such as teachers and salespersons. These are commercially available and can be conveniently used with hands-free microphones and manually adjustable transmitters. The sound amplification systems may help reduce vocal strain for professional speakers who need to address an audience in big or noisy locations, or who have difficulty projecting their voices in any environment. Amplifiers may also help reduce the phonasthenic symptoms of these patients.

BEHAVIOR READJUSTMENT VOICE THERAPY

The concept of "voice therapy" has matured during the last two decades. It has gained a well defined place in the voice disorder management armamentarium. It has become unchallengingly a part of the domain of the communication specialist (speech pathologist, logopedist, and phoniatrician). The procedures (methods) of voice therapy, variable as they may be, have gained support from qualitative clinical data, but now lack sufficient objective evidence for their mode of action and therapeutic efficacy.

Behavior readjustment voice therapy has developed primarily in response to the special situation of a patient with a dysphonic voice and a morphologically normal larynx that the laryngologist cannot modify by surgery or pharmacotherapy. The management of these cases was sought for in other nonconventional ways. Behavior readjustment voice therapy is the alternative. Thus, this type of voice therapy developed mainly to manage nonorganic (functional) voice disorders. A major salient feature of behavior readjustment voice therapy is that it encompasses two major domains: (1) counseling providing voice hygiene advice, and (2) exercises for the correction of faulty vocal techniques.

At present, a wide variety of "tools" for behavior readjustment voice therapy can be used for clinical trial with the voice patient. The voice clinician chooses the particular tool(s) most suited to each patient: mostly on subjective trial-and-error basis, supported by clinical experience to help determine which methods elicit a better or more easily produced voice. Although there are several known and recommended guidelines for the choice of a particular technique, there is still no conclusive evidence to decisively support one tool over another to "heal" a particular category of voice disorders. The ultimate choice of a "tool" for voice therapy is strongly influenced by the clinician's own theoretical biases about the structure and function of the vocal organ as well as the pathophysiological model of voice disorder. Some voice therapy programs concentrate mainly on voice hygiene advice, others on relaxation and breathing, and still others on pitch and loudness.

The Schools of Voice Therapy

The schools of voice therapy may be arbitrarily divided into five categories.

Specific Methods (Procedures)

Several voice therapy procedures directed towards the management of a particular vocal pathology may be grouped in this category. Some of these procedures can be a specific drill or maneuver. Others may offer an integrated therapy method, such as the pushing exercises resorted to in the management of paralytic dysphonia (Table 2–1).

Diverse Nonrelated Methods (Procedures)

This school of voice therapy does not postulate a particular general theory for the pathogenesis of disorders of voice. Instead, the clinician relies on his or her segmental analysis of the defective vocal and paravocal behaviors into elements specific to each patient. The clinician draws from an accumulated repertoire of facilitatory vocal drills believed to handle and correct the different defective elements of a vocal behavior. Defective vocal elements may range from excessive laryngeal muscular tension and muscular weakness, to pitch

Table 2–1. Management of specific disorders

Paralytic dysphonia	Pushing exercises*
Mutational dysphonia	Laryngeal position adujstment; lowering and pushing backward of the thyroid cartilage by manual manipulation and pressure**
Habitual/Psychological aphonia	Cough/hum, masking***

* From Froschels, Kastein, and Weiss (1955).
** From Aronson (1985)
*** From Boone (1988).

defects, faulty head or tongue position, and so on (Bastian & Nagorsky, 1987; Boone, 1988; Greene, 1980; Polow & Kaplan, 1986; Prater & Swift, 1987). This school usually gives plenty of time to voice hygiene advice (Boone, 1988; Johnson, 1985). The patient may be given certain tasks for application in daily life, as aids in helping the person to monitor and guard against voice abuse and misuse (Wilson, 1987). Hierarchial lists may be given to help the patient identify and avoid vocal stress situations (Boone, 1988).

Diverse Related Methods (Procedures)

Some voice clinicians, although remaining analytic in describing certain isolated defective elements (segments) of a vocal behavior as the basis for studying the nonorganic (functional) dysphonias, have tried to relate them to a dysfunction in a particular domain. Forchhammer (1974) ascribes the pathogenesis of the different types of nonorganic (functional) dysphonia to a variety of laryngeal muscular "insufficiencies." Sovijarvi (1974) relates all types of nonorganic (functional) dysphonias to "asymmetries" of the laryngeal cartilages. Those authors devised series of vocal drills to correct and "reverse" the insufficiencies or asymmetries they postulated as the cause of the dysphonia. (For further information regarding these methods of voice therapy consult Appendix 2.)

Holistic Methods (Procedures)

Few clinicians view the vocal pathology in a "gestalt" manner. They believe that voice production is an outcome of respiratory, phonatory, and articulatory activities occurring within a highly coordinated dynamic motor act framework. A defective voice may thus be envisaged as an outcome of an imbalance of this complex process of total communication. The therapy methods employed to correct a defective voice function usually adopt a holistic approach for restoring the balance of the respiratory, phonatory, and articulatory motor activities. Examples of the voice therapy methods that may fall under this heading are the chewing method of Froeschels (1952) and the Accent Method of Smith (Smith & Thyme, 1978).

Counseling

In some cases, no treatment or combination of treatments will achieve a satisfactory voice. Patients may then need counseling to learn how to live with a vocal deficit. The severity of the person's reaction to a problem determines whether it can be treated by a voice clinician or should be referred to a professional counselor. It is underscored that it is common for patients to become depressed because of their voice disorders and the need to modify their lives to accommodate.

REFERENCES

Arnold, G. E. (1962). Vocal rehabilitation of paralytic dysphonia. IX. Technique of intracordal injection. *Archives of Otolaryngology, 76*, 358.

Attaly, J. P., Gioux, M., Henry, C., Migueis, J., Ducourneau, A., & Triassac, L. (1990). Rehabilitation of abduction of the vocal cord by selective nerve anastomosis in dogs. *Review-Laryngology-Otology-Rhinology-Bord., 111*, (IV), 397.

Bastian, R. M., & Nagorsky, M. J. (1987). Laryngeal image biofeedback. *Laryngoscope, 97*, 1346.

Blitzer, A., & Brin, M. F. (1991). Laryngeal dystonia: A series with Botulinum toxin therapy. *Annals of Otology, Rhinology and Laryngology, 100*, 85.

Blom, E. D. (1978). The artificial larynx: Past and present. In S. J. Salmon & L. P. Goldstein (Eds.), *The artificial larynx handbook* (pp. 57–86). New York: Grune and Stratton, Inc.

Boone, D. R. (1988). *The voice and voice therapy* (4th ed.). Englewood Cliffs, NJ: Prentice-Hall.

Bouchayer, M., & Cornut, G. (1992). Micro surgical treatment of benign vocal fold lesions. Indications, technique, results. *Folia Phoniatrica* (Basel), *44*, 155.

Brodnitz, A. (1971). *Vocal rehabilitation* (4th ed.) Rochester, MN: American Academy of Ophthalmology and Otolaryngology.

Broman, H., Kotby, M. N., & Arlin, E. (1977, November). *Analysis of ten years laryngectomy. Material concerning adaptation and rehabilitation.* Paper presented at the first Middle East Cancer Conference, Cairo.

Brünings, W. (1911). Über eine neue Behandlungs Methode der Rekurrenslahmung. *Verhandlung das Vereins der Laryngologen, 18,* 583.

Burgess, L. P. A., & Yim, D. W. S. (1988). Thyroid cartilage flap reconstruction of the larynx following vertical partial laryngectomy: An interim report. *Laryngoscope, 98,* 605.

Dedo, H. H. (1976). Recurrent laryngeal nerve section for spastic dysphonia. *Annals of Otology, Rhinology & Laryngology, 85,* 451.

Enjell, H. (1984). *Assessment and treatment of vocal cord paralysis.* Unpublished doctoral thesis. Department of Otolaryngology. Sahlgren University Hospital, Gothenberg, Sweden.

Forchhammer, E. (1974). *Stemmens Funktioner og fejl funktioner.* Copenhagen, Denmark: Munksgaard.

Ford, C. N., & Bless, D. M. (1986). Clinical experience with injectable collagen for vocal fold augmentation. *Laryngoscope, 96,* 863.

Ford, C. N., Bless, D. M., & Lowery, J. D. (1991). Indirect laryngologic approach for injection of botulinum toxin in spasmodic dysphonia. *Otolaryngology, Head and Neck Surgery, 103*(5), 752.

Froeschels, E. (1952). Chewing method as therapy: A discussion with some philosophical conclusions. *Archives of Otolaryngology, 56,* 427.

Fukuda, F. (1970). Use of silicon injection in vocal rehabilitation. *Journal of Otolaryngology* (Fukuoka), *73,* 1506.

Greene, M. C. L. (1980). *The voice and its disorders* (4th ed.). Philadelphia: J. B. Lippincott.

Harris, T. M. (1992). The pharmacological treatment of voice disorders. *Folia Phoniatrica* (Basel), *44,* 143.

Hilgers, F. J. M., & Schouwenburg, P. F. (1990). A new low resistance, self-retaining prosthesis (Provox™) for voice rehabilitation after total laryngectomy. *Laryngoscope, 100,* 1202.

Hill, D. P., Meyers, A. D., & Harris, J. (1991). Autologous fat injection for vocal cord medialization in the canine larynx. *Laryngoscope, 101,* 344.

Hirano, M. (1975). Phonosurgery: Basic and clinical investigations. *Otologia* (Fukuoka), *21,* 239.

Hirano, M. (1976). Technique for glottic reconstruction following vertical partial laryngectomy: A preliminary report. *Annals of Otology, Rhinology & Laryngology, 85,* 25.

Isshiki, N. (1980). Recent advances in phonosurgery. *Folia Phoniatrica* (Basel), *32,* 119.

Isshiki, N., Tanabe, M., & Sawada, M. (1978). Arytenoid adduction for unilateral vocal cord paralysis. *Archives of Otolaryngology, 104,* 555.

Iwamura, S. (1986). Selective section of a thyroarytenoid branch of the recurrent laryngeal nerve for spastic dysphonia. In *Proceedings of 20th Congress of International Association of Logopedics and Phoniatrics (IALP),* p. 474. Tokyo.

Iwamura S., Tadiutchi K., Hosoya N., Tateoka H., & Fukayama S. (1986). Surgical treament for spastic dysphonia. *Journal of Otolaryngology* Japan, 89, 1422.

Johnson, T. S. (1985). *Vocal abuse reduction program*. San Diego: College-Hill Press.

King, B. T. (1939). A new and function restoring operation for bilateral abductor cord paralysis, preliminary report. *Journal of American Medical Association*, *112*, 814.

Kleinsasser, O. (1968). *Microlaryngoscopy and endolaryngeal microsurgery*. Toronto, Canada: W. B. Saunders Company.

Kleinsasser, O. (1991). Restoration of the voice in benign lesions of the vocal folds by endolaryngeal microsurgery. *Journal of Voice*, *5*(3), 257.

Kotby, M. N. (1986). Voice disorders: Recent diagnostic advances. *Egyptian Journal of Otolaryngology*, *3*(1), 69.

Miller, R. H., Woodson, G. E., & Jankovic, J. (1987). Botulinum toxin injection of the vocal fold for spasmodic dysphonia. *Archives of Otolaryngology*, *113*, 603.

Motta, G. (1984). *IL Laser A CO_2, Nella Microchirurgia Laringea*. Milano, Italy: Libreria Scientifica gia Ghedini s.r.l.

Ossaff R. H., Karlan M. S., & Sisson, G. A. (1983). Endoscopic laser arytenoidectomy. *Laser Surgery in Medicine*, *2*, 293.

Polow, N. G., & Kaplan, E. D. (1986). *Symptomatic voice therapy* (3rd ed.) San Diego, CA: College-Hill Press.

Prater, R. J., & Swift, R. W. (1987). *Manual of voice therapy* (3rd ed.). Boston: Little, Brown and Company.

Saito, S. (1977). Phonosurgery, basic study of the mechanism of phonation and endolaryngeal microsurgery. *Otologia (Fukuoka)*, *23*, 171.

Sato, F., & Ogura, J. (1978). Functional restoration for recurrent laryngeal paralysis. An experimental study. *Laryngoscope*, *88*, 855.

Schramm, V. L., May, M., & Lavorato, A. S. (1978). Gel foam paste injection for vocal fold paralysis: Temporary rehabilitation of glottic incompetence. *Laryngoscope*, *88*, 1268.

Singer, M. I. (1983). Tracheo-esophageal speech. Vocal rehabilitation after total laryngectomy. *Laryngoscope*, *93*, 1454.

Singer, M. I., & Blom, E. D. (1980). An endoscopic technique for restoration of voice after laryngectomy. *Annals of Otology, Rhinology & Laryngology*, *89*, 529.

Smith, S., & Thyme, K. (1978). *Accent metoden*. Herning: Special Paedagogisk Forlag.

Sovijarvi, A. (1974). *Therapeutic results of laryngeal asymmetric postures in dysphonic patients*. Tokyo: World Papers in Phonetics.

Sovijarvi, A. (1984). Some therapeutic exercises for rehabilitating functional dysphonias presented on videotape. In *The study of sounds, the proceedings of the Fourth World Congress of Phoneticians*, (Vol. XX) (pp. 445–457). Japan: The Phonetic Society of Japan.

Steiner, W. , Jaumann, M. P., & Pesch H. J. (1980). Endoskopische laserchirurgie in larynx. *Therapeutische Umschau / Revue Therapeutique*, *37*, 1103.

Takayama E., Fukuda H., Koawa N., & Saito S. (1988). A treatment for spastic dysphonia—Selective resection of the terminal branch of the recurrent laryngeal nerve in the thyroarytenoid muscle. *Journal of Japan Bronchoesophagological Society*, *39*,(3), 275.

Tucker, H. M. (1977). Reinnervation of the unilaterally paralyzed larynx. *Annals of Otology, Rhinology and Laryngology*, *86*, 789.

Van Lawrence, L. (1987). Common medications with laryngeal effects. *Ear, Nose, & Throat Journal*, *66*, 318.

von Leden, H., Yanagihara, N., & Wernre-Kukuk, E. (1967). Teflon in unilateral vocal cord paralysis. *Archives of Otolaryngology*, *85*, 110.

Wilson, D. K. (1987). *Voice problems of children* (3rd ed.). John Butler (Ed.). Baltimore: Williams and Wilkins.

CHAPTER 3

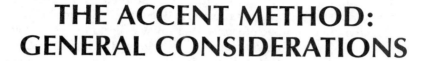

THE ACCENT METHOD: GENERAL CONSIDERATIONS

HISTORY

The Accent Method (AM) is a holistic process for voice therapy. It was developed by Svend Smith, a Danish speech therapist, speech scientist, and a phonetician in about 1936. Originally, Smith had developed this method to improve speech (stuttering) and voice. The Accent Method (AM) has an unfounded reputation of being an exotic method of therapy, because of the rich rhythms and body movements integral to the technique. In fact, it is a holistic approach to the treatment of voice.

When Smith began searching for an alternative tool to help speech and voice patients, the field was dominated by a general trend of employing static postural approaches to drills in general, whether articulatory (Forchhammer, 1927, as cited in Smith & Thyme, 1978), or general body movements as in Lingian gymnastics (Holmberg, 1939). Smith, on the other hand, envisioned verbal communication as a dynamic phenomenon from the begining. He was also convinced that intonation and stress (prosody) of speech were fundamental aspect of expressive communication. Similarly, Smith considered breathing as the prime excitor of the whole process of voice and speech production. These three aspects, dynamism, rhythmic intonation (accent), and expiratory breath control represent the fundamentals of the Accent Method (AM) of voice therapy.

Smith was searching for a rhythmic tool to develop, convey, and control the dynamic intonations (accent) of voice and speech production. He had been exposed to the rich and versatile West African drum rhythms accompanying Josephine Baker's singing. At the time, she was a regular star of the famous Tivoli Gardens in Copenhagen. Smith met Mr. Bogana, Mrs. Baker's drummer, and picked up the rhythms he thought relevant to what Smith was developing as the Accent Method (AM). Since then, these drum beats, though not essential for the Accent Method (AM), became a "trademark" for this therapeutic method (Smith & Thyme, 1978).

The dynamic approach to voice therapy was not completely novel when Smith started developing his technique. During the 1920s, Froeschels in Vienna started developing the chewing method for helping voice patients (Froeschels, 1943). A major aspect of that method is the dynamic association of several simultaneous phonatory and articulatory movements. These principles probably provided some inspiration to Svend Smith while he was developing the Accent Method (AM).

During the years since its introduction, the Accent Method (AM) has gained momentum from several basic studies related to phonetics (Smith & Thyme, 1978), physiology (Kotby, Shiromoto, & Hirano, 1993; Van den Berg, 1958), psychology and pedagology (Lauritzen, 1970), as well as clinical practice (Fex, Fex, Shiromoto, & Hirano, 1994; Kotby, El-Sady, Bassiouny, Abou-Rass, & Hegazi, 1991). These studies attempted to explain the rationale of the Accent Method (AM) and described its fundamentals and efficacy.

FUNDAMENTALS OF THE ACCENT METHOD

The Accent Method (AM) entails a dynamic integration of:

  A. Abdomino-diaphragmatic breathing.
  B. Accentuated rhythmic vowel play (phonation) and, later, articulation.
  C. Body and arm movements.

Despite the clear descriptive methodology and the well-defined basic rationale of the Accent Method (AM), many clinicians add additional details that personify their version of the method. There are, thus, many small variations of the fundamentals of Smith's Accent Method (AM).

Although vocal hygiene advice is not an integral part of the Accent Method (AM), a few guidelines are given to patients to ensure they do not damage their voices. Thus, one can still describe the Accent Method (AM) under the same general principles of behavioral readjustment voice therapy, in that it covers the two fundamental areas of:

1. Voice hygiene advice.
2. Correction of the faulty vocal technique.

Voice Hygiene Advice

Smith emphasized, contrary to what was the prevalent practice at his time, that no detailed explanation is given to the patient in the Accent Method (AM) about the nature of the voice pathology or what the Accent Method (AM) is doing to correct it. Following that paradigm, voice hygiene advice related to the Accent Method (AM) is rather limited. No detailed counseling is given about areas such as voice rest and anti-abuse tasks. Similarly, unduly long discussion of the patient's various psychological stresses is avoided.

Voice hygiene advice in connection with the Accent Method (AM) is rather simple and is often tailored to the direct needs of the patient. It is delivered in a way that makes it clear and easy to follow.

Two aspects related to voice hygiene, relaxation and vocal rest, need elaboration to clarify the way in which they are tackled in the practice of the Accent Method (AM).

Relaxation

Clinicians employing the Accent Method (AM) of voice therapy take note of the possible role of excessive tension in causing some vocal pathologies and in interfering with the management and the reversal of other pathologies. In the Accent Method (AM), however, no special devices or general body relaxation techniques are resorted to for the alleviation of excessive tension. Breathing exercises coordinated with the rhythmic dynamic body movements inherent to the Accent Method (AM) are the main tools used for achieving general relaxation. These exercises start at the very first stages of the therapy program.

The dynamic and activated movements of the articulators during the accent exercises help to relax the jaw, lips, and tongue; ease palatal movements; and widen the pharynx. The soft onset of phonation, producing a breathy voice, at the initial phases of the accent exercises alleviates hard glottal attacks that may be partially caused by increased muscular tension in the "larynx area." Faulty postures of the head, neck, and shoulders are usually corrected simultaneously with the dynamic body movements integrated with the rhythmic accent vocal exercises. Incorporation of these activities that reduce tension and invite relaxation via the general vocal exercises helps the clinician achieve relaxation in a time-efficient manner. The economic use of time becomes increasingly important as clinicians become more accountable to third-party payers and health care plans.

The general stresses and worries of the patient are given suitable attention, when needed. The increased self-confidence, which is usually nurtured by the Accent Method (AM), as well as the patient's experience of vocal improvement early in treatment may be as practical and as effective a tool in handling stress and worry as is counseling. The more difficult task of solving family, work, and personal conflicts of the tense patient is not a main objective of the Accent Method (AM) and is referred to professional counselors.

Voice Rest

Complete voice rest is not generally recommended. It is believed to be contraindicated in most chronic, nonorganic (functional), or organic voice disorders. In long-standing voice disorders, even with voice abuse/misuse forming an important predisposing factor, **complete** voice rest is not helpful. It may prove to be illogical and nonproductive; it is also difficult for the patient to accomplish, despite explanation and motivation; it may result in muscle atrophy and it may cause the patient to develop a phonophobia. In this respect, the clinician should not aim at training the patient to be "as silent as the sphinx."

Complete voice rest may be needed, however, for a limited length of time, following some acute voice problems, such as acute massive vocal trauma, acute physical trauma to the larynx involving the vocal folds, and extirpation surgery of the vocal fold. Complete voice rest is also recommended in cases of acute inflammation of the larynx (acute laryngitis).

Thus, voice hygiene advice in relation to the Accent Method (AM) can be classified into two simple categories:

    A. "Do–do not do" category.
    B. "Try to do" category.

"Do–Do Not Do" Category

The patient is urged to avoid only the behaviors of screaming, smoking, and alcohol consumption.

Screaming   Screaming is a major source of vocal trauma that may lead to such immediate effects as submucosal bleeding (Prater & Swift, 1987; Wilson, 1987) or to such more protracted effects as vocal nodules, polyps, and Reinke's edema. Screaming may also lead to exaggeration of the phonasthenic symptoms (Damsté & Lerman, 1975).

The clinician has, however, to explain to the patient that screaming can be of two types:

1. *Known, or conscious, screaming*, in which the patient is aware of its occurrence. An example of this type is how temperamental persons often communicate in daily life or what parents of young children may use to help discipline their offspring. Some professionals may need to indulge in this type of screaming to be heard, such as teachers in big, ill-prepared classrooms, salespeople, and, sometimes, stage actors.

2. *Unknown, or unconscious, screaming*, although less easily appreciated, is sometimes more injurious for voice. An example of this vocal malpractice is speaking against a loud background noise as in moving cars, trains, and planes. One may also indulge in such "screaming speaking" while in confined places with loud music or with many people talking loudly as in cocktail parties or noisy restaurants.

   The importance of dealing with this type of screaming is that a patient is not aware that he or she is abusing the voice during such an activity. The patient may be aware of its after-effects through increase of the vocal symptoms. This type of screaming can be more easily avoided than the known (conscious) type. Screaming is usually not a practice required to conduct daily life. The clinician is, thus, asking the patient to quit an unneeded behavior. Contrary to absolute voice rest, such advice is expected to be followed by the patient. In cases in which the patient is obliged to phonate loudly, as when addressing big groups of listeners or as when forced to speak in noisy places, alternative devices can be recommended. This may include the use of a whistle by parents to get the attention of their children; the use of amplifiers and microphones by public speakers, teachers, and salespeople; talking to people no further away than an arm's distance; and making modification to environments for more vocal hygienics.

Smoking   Smoking has been shown to have an ill effect on the vocal fold mucosa (Auerbach, Hammond, & Carfinkel, 1970). Clinical and histopathological evidence is abundant. Smoking is a known predisposing factor in the causation of laryngeal cancer, dysplasia (Auerbach et al., 1970), Reinke's edema (Fritzell & Hertegard, 1984), and other minimal associated pathological lesions (MAPLs), as well as nonorganic (functional) dysphonia.

The patient is instructed to stop "active" smoking, which is a form of voluntary self-inflicting laryngeal damage. The patient should be also instructed to avoid "passive" smoking, in which there is exposure to other peoples' smoking. It is sad to point out that in many parts of the world the human rights of nonsmokers are not strictly observed. Passive smoking can be injurious (Stell & Watt, 1984; Stock, 1980). Equally disappointing is that most smokers cannot or will not comply with the request to ease smoking. This failure has a direct impact on the outcome of treatment.

Alcoholic Beverages (Spirits)   The negative effects of spirits on voice can be multifactorial:

1. Strong liquors may cause pharyngeal and reflex laryngeal congestion, increasing the vascularity of the vocal fold mucosa and may thus make the surface more vulnerable to microhematomas in response to vocal trauma (Flanders & Rothman, 1982).
2. People tend to speak more loudly and more freely under the effect of alcohol, thus increasing the possibility of vocal abuse.
3. The unhealthy symbiosis of alcohol and smoking is rather common and a synergistic effect has been directly linked to laryngeal carcinoma.

"Try to Do" Category"

The patient is encouraged to develop a positive attitude toward voice and the larynx by observing certain hygienic practices.

Increase Fluid Intake   Sufficient hydration of the body leads to the production of thin watery secretions from the mucous and mixed glands of the mucosa of the larynx and trachea. This type of secretion is easy to expel by coughing. Thick tenacious secretions, on the other hand, tend to stay and linger over the vocal fold mucosa, giving the patient the feeling of "a veil over the voice," or a sticky "mucus" over the vocal fold, that has to be expelled. The patient usually achieves that by repeated, sometimes violent hawking and clearing of the throat. This hawking may cause trauma to the vocal fold mucosa.

The advice to overhydrate, by excessive fluid intake, helps to guarantee the production of more watery secretions in patients who suffer from a tendency to accumulation of thick tenacious secretions. The absolute amount of fluid in terms of liters per day is difficult to state. The amount varies depending on weather conditions (heat and humidity), and on individual metabolic needs. The recommended fluid intake should be sufficient to produce plenty of pale-colored, diluted urine, indicating successful overhydration (Van Lawrence, 1987). The type of fluid may include water, milk, fruit juices, and other simple noncaffeinated beverages.

Patients are sometimes over-concerned about the effect of foods and drinks on their voices. At this stage, they usually tend to ask the clinician about what they should avoid. The patient can usually be reassured that there are no additional dietary restrictions unless he or she has esophageal reflux. Avoidance of very spicy foods as well as foods and drinks with extreme temperatures may, however, be advised.

Hawking Avoidance   Attempts to clear the throat from sticky secretions are related to the previous point. Hawking is a potential source of vocal trauma, as it entails vigorous banging and friction of the vocal folds. It may temporarily rid the patient of such secretions, but it tends to increase the secretions of the thick, sticky sort of mucus. Throat clearing may thus lead to the initiation of a vicious circle. Abstinence from such hawking may break the circle. Recommendations of soft open coughing with a big rush of expiratory air is thought to help the patient avoid a feeling of a sticky secretion causing "veiling the voice." Such a maneuver is difficult to carry out and is often not effective in achieving its goal. Overhydration by increased fluid intake (thus producing less tenacious and less sticky secretion) may, on the other hand, help to ease this symptom and break the vicious circle.

The aformentioned voice hygiene advice is briefly described to the patient during the preliminary session, in which rapport is being built between the patient and the clinician. As a general final remark, the patient is encouraged to lead a "healthy" life, including good regular sleep, well-balanced diet, adequate sports or physical activity, good care of the teeth, skin, and chest, and care of the bowel habit (Brodnitz, 1971).

Correction of Faulty Vocal Habits

Accent Method (AM) exercises aim at improving voice and speech production. Accent Method (AM) does not deal with particular isolated defective aspects of voice such as pitch or loudness. Rather, it aims in a holistic manner at a better balance between excitor and vibrator, in other words between expiratory phonatory air flow (rate, force, and velocity) and vocal fold muscle power (adductory force). Accent Method (AM) exercises further aim at establishing better coordination of the voice produced at the glottis and the resonatory articulatory activities. It thus improves such final aspects of speech production as projection, sonority, and prosody through indirect work on coordination. For the technical details of the methodology of the Accent Method (AM), see Chapter 4.

Rationale and Mode of Action

Voice physiology research in the 1950s stressed the importance of the expiratory air flow at the glottis in voice production (Smith, 1954). The aerodynamic myoelastic theory of voice production (Van den Berg, 1958) ascribed a key role for the Bernoulli effect at the glottis in maintaining the vibratory motion of the vocal fold mucosa. Despite recent introduction of other factors (Titze, 1986, 1991), aerodynamic events at and around the glottis, including the Bernoulli effect, play a crucial role in voice production and in maintaining a good symmetrical vibratory mucosal wave cycle.

    These observations led Smith to stress the importance of breath control as the key to the enhancement of the Bernoulli effect at the glottis. Accordingly, he developed the accent exercises of the Accent Method (AM) using abdomino-diaphragmatic accentuated rhythmic expiratory pulses (Smith & Thyme, 1978).

    Smith's original hypothesis (1954) postulated that respiratory support is the key to the proper production of the accent exercises and, hence, to voice improvement. In testing this hypothesis, Kotby et al.(1993) have carried out a study on three subjects with varying degrees of training with the Accent Method (AM). In these subjects, there was a clear increase of the air flow through the glottis in response to the accentuated vocal utterances (accent exercises). This was accompanied by simultaneous increase in the sound pressure level (SPL) and fundamental frequency (F_0) (Figure 3–1). These observations support the notion that the key to the adjustment of the vocal parameters in the accent exercises may be the increased glottal air flow in response to the accentuated abdomino-diaphragmatic expiratory pulses. The increase in SPL can be explained by the increased air flow causing increase in subglottal pressure (Psub). The increase in F_0, however, may be a response to the increased Psub (Titze, 1989). The increase in F_0 was, however, bigger than expected from the increased Psub. It is suggested that the accent exercises may be associated with activation of the cricothyroid muscle, with the resultant extra rise in F_0. The study

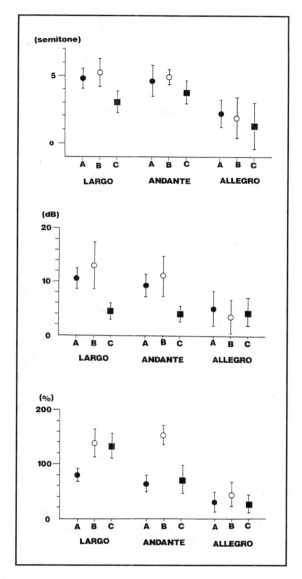

Figure 3–1. Mean ± SD for increase in fundamental frequency (ΔF_0) (in semitones) (top), sound pressure level (ΔSPL) (in dB) (middle), and air flow rate (ΔU) (in percentage increase) (bottom) for three subjects (A, B, and C) and the three tempos.

also demonstrated that the trained persons showed higher increases of SPL and F_0 in response to increased glottic air flow. It showed also that with increased training persons use the increase in air flow to effect the rise in SPL and F_0 more efficiently.

Further studies using other approaches are needed to provide a more complete explanation of the mode of action of the Accent Method (AM) in correcting faulty vocal behavior.

Mode of Action   The Accent method (AM) is described as managing two opposing functional deficits—a state of excessive glottal waste, and a state of excessive glottic tightness.

In cases of vocal fold paralysis with loss of muscle tone and persistence of a phonatory gap, the enhanced air flow in response to the accent exercises can produce an aerodynamic adductory (suction) effect that will help a small glottal gap (waste) to close despite the paralysis. The relaxed crescendo increase in air flow does not usually lead to a marked increase in the subglottic pressure. This is a beneficial effect that may guard against blowing the paretic folds apart with resultant voice breaks (Dalhoff & Kitzing, 1987).

In case of hyperfunctional dysphonia with excessive adductory muscle force, the vocal fold mucosal wave is impeded because of the tightness of the glottis. The accent exercises help to augment and accelerate the phonatory expiratory air flow in a gradual crescendo, providing optimal medially directed forces (suction) that help to approximate the vocal folds without the need for extra sphincteric activity of the muscles (Lauritzen, 1970). In this respect, the improved timing between the exhaled air and the onset of phonatory coaptation of the vocal folds achieved by the accent exercises helps also to reduce the tendency toward muscular hyperfunction.

The Accent Method (AM) does not focus on isolated drills to correct pitch or loudness. Through the restoration of the physiological balance among the flow, Psub, and laryngeal muscle contractions, the optimal habitual and comfortable pitch usually emerges. Excessive loudness, on the other hand, is corrected through the accent exercises easing muscular hyperfunction. The dynamic range of voice intensity is enhanced by the loudness variations during the accent exercises.

The Accent Method (AM) may be used for the management of selected voice and speech prosody disorders.

Indications for The Accent Method in Voice Disorder Management

In the treatment of voice disorders, the Accent Method (AM) may be used as the main therapeutic line or it may supplement such other treatment as phonosurgery or pharmacotherapy.

Mainstream Therapy   This is indicated in the management of some organic lesions and MAPLs as well as most of the nonorganic (functional) voice disorders.

Organic Voice Disorders   Organic voice disorders subject to Accent Method (AM) management include:

1. Paralytic dysphonia with disordered mobility of one or both vocal folds leaving a phonatory glottal gap of about 1–2 mm. Larger gaps usually need additional preliminary surgical procedures (Kotby et al., 1991).
2. Paralysis of the vocal folds resulting in persistent glottal stenosis that does not need urgent surgical intervention. The voice in this condition, though essentially free, may manifest a mild strained character. The Accent Method (AM), with its respiratory and phonatory exercises, may help to ease the voice problem and may improve the respiratory difficulty by relaxing the tensely adducted vocal folds.
3. Paralytic dysphonia when the superior laryngeal nerve is affected, causing a phonatory problem that may affect pitch control.
4. The Accent Method (AM) may be utilized to ease the phonatory hyperfunction in patients with dysplasia. After the removal of the dysplastic patch for histological examination, voice therapy is introduced as a major element in eliminating and easing phonatory hyperfunction, which is an important predisposing factor of dysplasia. Voice therapy helps also to improve the dysphonic voice of the patient.
5. As a primary treatment for sulcus glottideus is not universally agreed on, the use of noninvasive voice therapy may be indicated as the first possibility in intervention. The results of voice therapy for this condition are, however, not very promising. Voice therapy may help reduce the phonatory gap and ease the stiffness of the mucosa.
6. In cases of dysphonia due to iatrogenic effect of hormonal therapy leading to vocal muscularization lowering the pitch of the female voice, the Accent Method (AM) is used to help the patient adapt to the new anatomical changes (increased

mass of the vocal folds) and "find" an alternative optimal pitch and eliminating any possible emerging faulty vocal compensatory behavior.

7. Traumatic conditions managed by the Accent Method (AM) can include acute vocal trauma which is usually managed by voice rest. Soft, breathy accent exercises can assist in easing the condition and helping accelerate the patient's return to normal vocal activities. Also, the Accent Method (AM) is useful in unresolved attacks of bronchitis with protracted coughing episodes that lead to hyperirritability of the larynx and increased susceptibility to laryngeal spasms. The voice may also acquire strained character. Soft, breathy accent exercises may break this vicious circle by reducing the irritability of the larynx and improving voice quality.

8. Acute laryngitis in professional voice users may be helped by the Accent Method (AM), emphasizing use of very soft onset phonation. Short, repeated exercises several times a day during the acute phase are an appropriate choice.

Nonorganic (Functional) Voice Disorders   The Accent Method (AM) is indicated for:

1. All subtypes of the habitual nonorganic (functional) voice disorders; the Accent Method (AM) is a satisfactory selection as the main primary line of therapy.
2. The Accent Method (AM) has proved to be suitable for managing carefully selected cases of childhood hyperfunctional dysphonia.
3. Ventricular dysphonia, with no real hypertrophy of the ventricular bands, is well managed by the Accent Method (AM) of voice therapy, alone.
4. After the return of voice in cases of habitual aphonia, utilizing a series of specific vocal exercises (see Chapter 2), the patient may be helped by a brief Accent Method (AM) therapy program. The accent exercises stabilize the newly "rediscovered" voice.
5. Psychogenic voice disorders with bizarre vocal behavior are also usually managed by the Accent Method (AM) of voice therapy. In some cases, psychiatric treatment is also needed.

Minimal Associated Pathological Lesions (MAPLs)   MAPLs amenable to the Accent Method (AM) are:

1. Small soft vocal nodules in adults are effectively and satisfactorily treated by the Accent Method (AM) of voice therapy.
2. Contact granuloma is well managed by a prolonged program of voice therapy utilizing the Accent Method (AM).
3. Early Reinke's edema with a limited involvement of the vocal fold may be reversed by a well planned accent therapy program.

Vocal Problems of Professional Voice Users   The Accent Method (AM) has a definite place in the management of professional voice problems. The accent exercises may help the singing voice by:

- Providing an optimal physiological basis for voice production.
- Eliminating faulty mechanisms of voice production.

The accent exercises do not, however, modify the esthetics of the singing voice. These particular aspects need the help of a singing teacher.

Supplementary Therapy   The Accent Method (AM) may be used to supplement such other lines of therapy as phonosurgery or pharmacotherapy. This supplementary therapy is thought to be beneficial by achieving the goals:

- Eliminating predisposing faulty vocal habits to avoid recurrence.
- Acquainting the patient with the newly adjusted vocal apparatus to make maximal use of the potential vocal improvement.

Examples in which the Accent Method (AM) may be utilized as an adjuvent line of therapy include the following:

1. Voice therapy may be given preoperatively or may actively begin 1 week after phonosurgery—especially when surgical correction necessitates a major morphological derangement (as advanced Reinke's edema), or if surgical management of the laryngeal pathology (as in malignant lesions) is apt to leave a permanent anatomical defect.
2. Accent exercises may be given simultaneously with radiotherapy for glottic cancer to alleviate the acute voice problems caused by radiotherapy, and to avoid permanent vocal derangements and improve the final vocal results (Fex & Henriksson, 1970).
3. The aftermath of correction and reconstruction following various types of physical trauma to the larynx may be eased out by a well planned accent therapy program.

4. In selected cases of reconstruction following partial laryngectomy, accent exercises may improve the "residual" voice
by helping the coaptation of the newly reconstructed "glottis" and enhance loudness.
5. Spasmodic dysphonia (SD) is usually treated by an initial surgical intervention (nerve resection or Botulinum toxin A injection)
aimed at reducing the hyperadductory tendency in adductor SD.
The Accent Method (AM) can be utilized to maximize the vocal
improvement following surgery and to alleviate the breathy voice
resulting from possible postoperative phonatory waste.

Indications for the Accent Method in Speech Disorder Management

Dysarthria (Sy. dysarthrophonia)   In dysarthria, a breakdown in
speech and voice, dysprosody may be one of the main factors reducing overall speech intelligibility. The rhythmic accentuations of the
Accent Method (AM) directly help to improve prosody and voice.
The improved breath control helps also to reduce the labored nature of the dysarthric speech.

Stuttering   The improvement of the integrated rhythmic respiratory, phonatory, and articulatory activities together with dynamic body and limb movements in response to the Accent exercises
may lead to improvement of fluency and reduction of the manifestations of struggle in stuttering.

The Accent Method in Prosody Disorders

Delayed or deviant development of language may affect several lin-
guistic and paralinguistic domains. Dysprosody, which may be a
manifestation of delayed language development, can be improved
by the rhythmic accentuations of the Accent Method (AM). These
exercises, besides being agreeable to children, improve associative
body movement that may be affected as part of the syndrome of
delayed language development. These rhythmic accentuations are
especially beneficial in building up a quasinormal prosody in the
speech of children who are hearing impaired.

REFERENCES

Auerbach, O., Hammond, E. C., & Carfinkel, L. (1970). Histological changes
in the larynx in relation to smoking habits. *Journal of Cancer, 25,* 92.

Brodnitz, F. S., (1971). *Vocal rehabilitation* (4th ed.). Rochester, MN: American Academy of Ophthalmology and Otolaryngology.

Dalhoff, K., & Kitzing, P. (1987). Voice therapy according to Smith comments on the Accent Method to treat disorders of voice and speech. *Journal of Research in Singing and Applied Vocal Pedagogy, 11*(1), 15.

Damsté, A. H., & Lerman, J. W. (1975). *An introduction to voice pathology.* Springfield, IL: Charles C. Thomas.

Fex, S., & Henriksson, B. (1970). Phoniatric treatment combined with radiotherapy of laryngeal cancer for the avoidance of radiation damage. *Acta Otolaryngologica* (Stockholm), (Suppl.), *263*, 128.

Fex, B., Fex, S., Shiromoto, O., & Hirano, M. (1994). Acoustic analysis of functional dysphonia before and after voice therapy (Accent Method). *Journal of Voice, 7*(4), 163.

Flanders, W. D., & Rothman, K. J. (1982). Interaction of alcohol and tobacco in laryngeal cancer. *American Journal of Epidemiology, 115*, 371.

Fritzell, B., & Hertegard, S. (1984). A retrospective study of treatment for vocal fold edema: A preliminary report. In J. A. Kirchner (Ed.), *Vocal fold histopathology, a symposium.* (pp. 57–64). San Diego, CA: College-Hill Press.

Froeschels, E. (1943). Hygiene of voice. *Archives of Otolaryngology, 38*, 122.

Holmberg, O. (1939). *Den svenska gymnastikens utvekling. Per Henrik Ling och hans yrke.* Stockholm: Natur Och Kultur.

Kotby, M. N., El-Sady, S. R., Bassiouny, S. E., Abou- Rass, Y. A., & Hegazi, M. A. (1991). Efficacy of the Accent Method of voice therapy. *Journal of Voice, 5*(4), 316.

Kotby, M. N., Shiromoto, O., & Hirano, M. (1993). The Accent Method of voice therapy: Effect of accentuations on F_0, SPL and air flow. *Journal of Voice, 7*(2), 319.

Lauritzen, K. (1970). Om Taleundervisning efter accentmetoden. *Medlemsblad for Talepaedagogisk Forening, 6*, 132.

Prater, R. J., & Swift, R. W. (1987). *Manual of voice therapy* (3rd ed.). Boston: Little, Brown and Co.

Smith, S. (1954). Remarks on the physiology of the vibrations of the vocal cords. *Folia Phoniatrica* (Basel), 6, 166.

Smith, S., & Thyme, K. (1978). *Accent Metoden.* Herning: Special Paedagogisk Forlag.

Stell, P. M., & Watt, J. (1984). Squamous metaplasia of the subglottic space and its relation to smoking. *Annals of Otology, Rhinology & Laryngology, 93*, 124.

Stock, S. L. (1980). Risks the passive smoker runs. *Lancet, 2*(8203), 1082.

Titze, I. R. (1986). Mean intraglottic pressure in vocal fold oscillation. *Journal of Phonetics, 14*, 359.

Titze, I. R. (1989). On the relation between subglottal pressure and fundamental frequency in phonation. *Journal of the Acoustic Society of America, 85*(2), 901.

Titze, I. R. (1991). Phonation threshold pressure: A missing link in glottal aerodynamics. *NCVS Status and Progress Report*-1, June, 1.

Van den Berg, J. W. (1958). Myoelastic aerodynamic theory of voice pro-
    duction. *Journal of Speech and Hearing Research, 1*(3), 227.
Van Lawrence, L. (1987). Common medications with laryngeal effects. *Ear
    Nose and Throat Journal, 66*, 318.
Wilson, D. K. (1987). *Voice problems of children* (3rd ed.). Baltimore:
    Williams & Wilkins.

CHAPTER 4

■

THE ACCENT METHOD: TECHNICAL CONSIDERATIONS

ESTABLISHING RAPPORT

Discussions of technical considerations appropriately begin with a discussion of rapport. Rapport establishes the relationship between clinicians and patients and sets the tone for subsequent treatment. Smith has stressed the critical importance of creating a clinical atmosphere of equality and friendship between the clinician and the patient, rather than an authoritarian classroom atmosphere of an instructor/pupil relationship (Smith & Thyme, 1978). Smith strongly recommends the clinician avoid being too critical about vocal defects and stresses the need to build the patient's self-confidence by reinforcing his or her positive skills. Without positive rewards, the patient may become self-conscious about defects of voice and, in attempting to correct the defects, develop unwanted compensatory tension.

Contrary to the prevalent trend when the Accent Method (AM) was formulated, Smith discourages clinicians from providing detailed explanations of the principles of the technique or the physiology/pathology of voice production. It is his thought that instructions are tedious and confuse a patient more than help him or her learn new ways to use the anatomical structure to produce a relaxed healthy voice.

Smith does, however, invest considerable time in understanding the patient's subjective complaint and its impact on his or her daily and professional life. This is thought to be important, even in the presence of a detailed referral. Listening to patients' complaints related to voice and to life, in general, helps build a good rapport between the clinician and the patient and helps the clinician appreciate the sources of stress related to voice production. This "venti-lation" of the patient's problems in the presence of an expert atten-tive and supportive ear may also help to ease a patient's tension. Listening to patient complaints is not unique to the Accent Method (AM), as it is considered central to most treatment programs.

Contrary to the Accent Method (AM) underlying philosophy that detailed patient instructions should be avoided, the Accent Method (AM) treatment plan begins with an explanation to justify starting with breathing exercises for a patient with a throat or voice problem and no complaint of breathing difficulties. This is not difficult for the patient to understand when clinicians present a simple explanation of voice production using an analogy between the "car-motor/gasoline" and "vocal folds/breathing." Voice is pro-duced in the voice box (larynx), which correlates to the "car-motor." To have control of the "motor," one must have control of the "gaso-line pedal." The gasoline is like the expiratory air in voice produc-tion. Breathing is necessary to "drive" voice production, as gasoline is essential to "drive" the car motor. Thus, it is natural to work on better breath control to achieve better control of the "voice box" and modify its problems.

The clinician may also explain and point out that the abdomi-no-diaphragmatic type of breathing may be more suited for phona-tory purposes, as it facilitates using larger amounts of air. More importantly, in abdomino-diaphragmatic breathing, the expiratory air flow is enhanced by support of the abdominal muscles. An addi-tional gain from turning the breathing mode from upper chest (clavicular) to abdominal diaphragmatic is the possible reduction of activity of the accessory respiratory neck and shoulder muscles, which, in turn, may reduce some laryngeal tension and aberrant voice production.

With this brief explanation and stress of the importance of breathing to voice production and the direct relation of breath con-trol to the patient's complaint, the clinician has prepared the pa-tient for the next step, direct breathing exercises.

BREATHING EXERCISES

Importance

The necessity of training breathing for the management of voice disorders is not universally accepted (Boone, 1988). In light of the generally accepted theory of phonation, namely the aerodynamic myoelastic theory, the role of expiratory air flow in voice production cannot be minimized, and its role in treatment should be readily understood by clinicians treating voice disorders.

The Accent Method (AM) of voice therapy places an unequivocal importance on the training of breathing: It is considered to be the fundamental basis of this holistic method of voice therapy. The basic preliminary phase of direct respiratory or breathing exercises stresses acquiring abdomino-diaphragmatic breathing at rest. Subsequent phases carry this acquisition through to conversational speech.

Abdominal expiratory support has been stressed by several clinicians as an important facilitatory procedure in voice therapy (Forchhammer, 1974; Smith & Thyme, 1978). The procedures to achieve this goal differ considerably. Most clinicians work mainly with the muscles of the anterior abdominal wall, which activate simultaneously with the flank muscles (oblique and transverse abdominal muscles), for expiratory support. Few clinicians have claimed to train the lumbar back muscles to participate in expiratory support in their voice therapy techiques (Forchhammer, 1974). Coactivation of the abdominal and flank muscles is, however, the main target of the expiratory exercises used in the Accent Method (AM). These exercises are effective in reaching the goals of better respiratory support and are rather easy to convey clinically to the patient.

Breathing for Biological Needs Versus for Communicative Purposes

Clinicians are advised at this stage to outline the main characteristics and differences of breathing for biological needs and breathing for voice and speech production. Quiet breathing for biological needs is a cyclic phenomena that has a relatively short and shallow inspiratory phase followed by an expiratory phase of an equal length. There is usually no pause between inspiration and expiration at rest, although a short pause follows the expiratory phase before the next cycle starts (Figure 4–1A). Under basic resting conditions, this cycle is repeated 14–16 times per minute. Quiet breathing for biological needs, which occupies the greater part of respiratory activities, is usually nasal. Nasal breathing warms and filters the air before it reaches the lungs.

Breathing for communicative purposes, voice and speech production, is distinctively different from the aforementioned type of breathing. It is usually formed of a quick deep inspiration followed immediately by a long phasic expiration that varies in length, depending on the length of the phrase and the type and distribution of stressed syllables (Greene, 1980; Luchsinger & Arnold, 1965) (Figure 4–1B). The large amount of air needed during the rapid inspiration cannot be supplied by nasal breathing alone. Breathing for communicative purposes is usually both oral and nasal (oro-nasal). This oronasal breathing helps regulate the needed air supply without causing any audible noises that would detract from the message being delivered by the speaker.

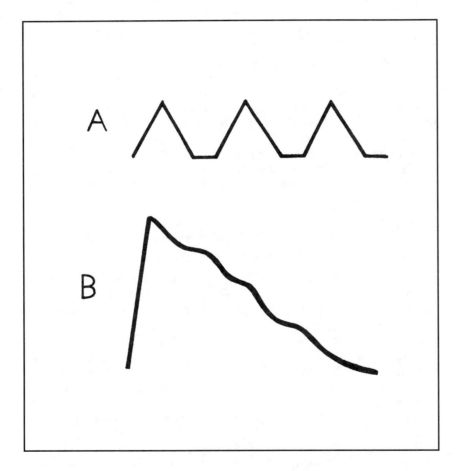

Figure 4–1. The respiratory cycle in (A) Quiet breathing for biological needs and (B) Quick, deep inspiration followed by a long phasic expiration in voice and speech production.

Abdomino-Diaphragmatic Breathing

Breathing exercises preparatory to voice readjustment aims at acquiring abdomino-diaphragmatic breathing. Compared to upper chest breathing, abdomino-diaphragmatic breathing is thought to have advantages that facilitate subsequent accent voice exercises:

A. **It allows the exchange of bigger volumes** of air during the respiratory cycle, thus reducing the respiratory rate. It allows also the production of a longer expiratory air stream.

B. **It reduces extra tension in the neck and shoulder muscles** that can be caused by the activation of the accessory respiratory muscles used in upper chest or clavicular breathing.

C. **It allows the patient to have a better control of the expiratory pulmonary pulses** that represent the driving force of the self-sustained vibratory vocal fold movements.

D. With the better control of expiratory air, **it allows a better chance for a more proper timing between exhalation and the onset of phonation,** an important prerequisite for "good" voice production.

E. It moves the focus away from the larynx GNP on to the respiratory system in much the same way tone focus or resonance balance exercises move the focus to the face resonators.

F. This rhythmic, quiet, and relatively deep cyclic breathing **helps to ensure general relaxation and alleviation of unnecessary tension.** This goal can be helped by starting breathing exercises in the recumbent position, thus maximizing this relaxation effect. In the recumbent position, the anterior abdominal wall is free to move up and down with the abdomino-diaphragmatic breathing and forces of gravity. Although the action of the diaphragm and gravital forces on the breathing pattern in the supine and upright position differ significantly, beginning in the supine position not only improves relaxation, it also heightens the patient's awareness of the role the abdomen can play in breathing and sound production. The breathing exercises are then and, as soon as possible, practiced in the sitting position to acquire the same relaxation effect in a more practical posture for voice and speech production.

Training Procedure

Classically, the patient is asked to lie supine on a relatively firm couch. A pillow under the knee may help to relax the abdominal muscles. In the recumbent (supine) position, the chest cage and the shoulders are resting on the couch and are not allowed to move. In this position, the abdominal wall is allowed, on the other hand, to move freely up and down with the rhythmic abdomino-diaphragmatic breathing. It is important to ensure that the upper chest and shoulders are **resting** and relaxing, with all respiratory efforts transferred to the abdominal level (Lauritzen, 1970). Awareness of the abdominal wall movement is heightened by placing a book on the abdomen. The book rides up and down with the abdominal movement and serves as an indicator of respiratory displacement (Figure 4–2). While in supine position the patient is asked to breathe freely and quietly through a slightly opened mouth and the nose. The patient is told to move the air in and out with as little resis-

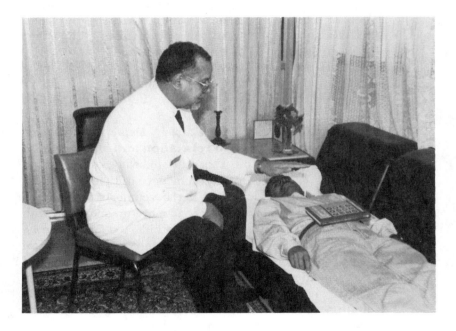

Figure 4–2. Breathing exercises in recumbent position. A book is put on the abdomen to illustrate the abdominal wall movements during breathing.

tance as possible. There should be no audible noise. Once the patient finds this task easy, the individual is moved to the next stage of treatment.

Now, instead of the book, the patient is asked to put a hand on the abdominal wall and feel its free movement with breathing. This hand acts only as a guide and does not help to push the abdominal wall inward with expiration. It is usually possible within a short period of time, even within the first training session, for the patient to acquire this type of abdomino-diaphragmatic breathing. Once the patient has managed this abdomino-diaphragmatic breathing and has the feeling of the abdominal muscle movement in relation to the respiratory cycle, the patient is asked to sit in an ordinary chair. With the hand on the abdomen, the patient is asked to breathe again freely through the nose and mouth and feel the abdominal wall movement outward and inward in response to abdominal inspiration and expiration, respectively (Figure 4–3). Rate of breathing and expiration phase length is varied. The clini-

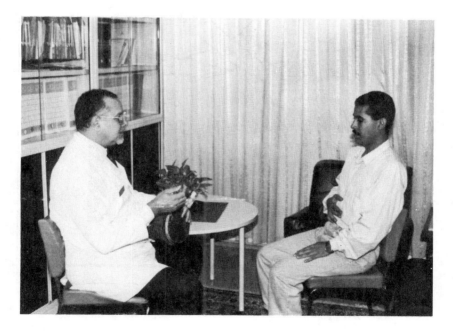

Figure 4–3. After the patient has mastered the abdomino-diaphragmatic breathing in the sitting position, the rhythmic phonatory exercises are initiated and practiced.

cian uses hand signals and table taps to help the patient follow the breathing movements and tempo. Most patients can acquire this type of breathing in **both the supine and sitting** position in the first therapeutic session.

If the patient fails to acquire these movements smoothly, the patient is asked to put the back of the hand on the abdominal wall of the clinician to feel his or her abdominal wall movements (outward and inward) in response to breathing (Figure 4–4). In this

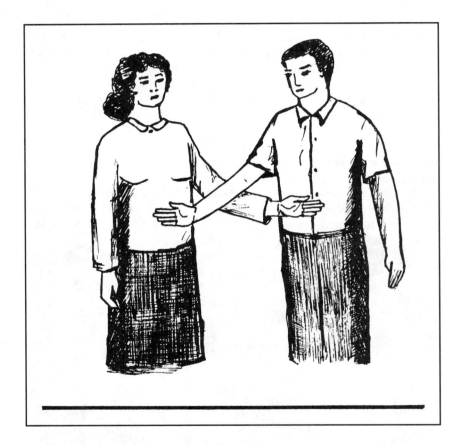

Figure 4–4. The patient is asked to put the back of the hand on the abdominal wall of the clinician to feel his or her abdominal wall movements (outward and inward) in response to breathing. This facilitates acquisition of the abdomino-diaphragmatic breathing in patients who have not responded to the supine-book exercise.

way the hand of the patient can **feel** the rhythmic contractions of the abdominal muscles. This maneuver is helpful in giving the patient an idea about what is supposed to happen in this type of respiratory maneuver. Feeling the clinician's movements is more effective than either providing theoretical verbal explanations or repeating the supine and sitting trials the patient has already failed to integrate. In few, extra rigid patients abdomino-diaphragmatic breathing may be acquired by trying it in the recumbent left or right **lateral** position.

When the abdomino-diaphragmatic breathing has been mastered by the patient in the sitting position, it can be attempted in the standing position (Figure 4–5). In this position, a swaying body movement can be added to the in/expiratory movements, following the rhythmic abdomino-diaphragmatic breathing. The patient is asked to stand with the feet slightly apart, with one foot in a slightly forward position to facilitate and stabilize the swaying movements. Forward movements are coupled with inspiration and backward movement with expiration.

Breathing exercises are usually easily managed by the voice clinician. For a very few extraordinary patients who are resistant to treatment, help of the physiotherapist may be necessary.

The slow, deep abdomino-diaphragmatic breathing trained in this phase of the therapy program allows the patient to experience suitable pauses in between the respiratory cycles. The slow rate of breathing with better pausing prepares the patient to utilize this optimally during the rhythmic vocal exercises in the subsequent phases of the Accent Method (AM) program. It should be stressed that one of the ultimate goals of the Accent Method (AM) is improved phrasing with optimal speech rate (Lauritzen, 1970).

PHONATORY EXERCISES

Preparatory Phase (Prephonatory Phase)

As soon as the abdomino-diaphragmatic breathing is mastered, a sound is added to the expiratory phase. The first such sound is an unvoiced fricative /f/. The patient is asked to feel the mild resistance to the air flow at the lips and is asked to produce a long unstressed sound throughout the expiratory phase (Figure 4–6). The sounds /s/ and /ʃ/ are then tried in a similar manner. When this associative respiratory articulatory activity is mastered, the patient is asked to produce these same sounds with an accentuated

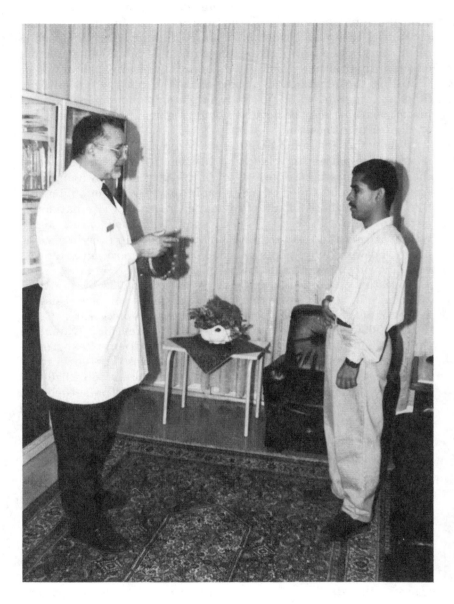

Figure 4–5. The respiratory and later the phonatory rhythmic exercises are transferred to the standing position. Associated body and arm movements can be practiced more freely while standing.

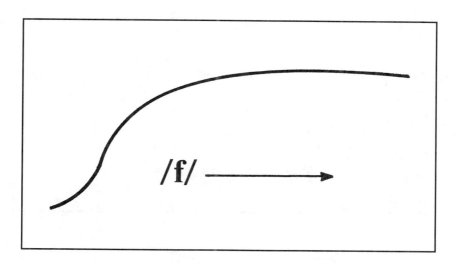

Figure 4–6. A prolonged expiration producing the nonvoiced /f/ sound to help the patient perceive the resistance to expiratory air flow at the lips.

final segment (Figure 4–7). The expiratory utterance will take the form of a short, soft segment followed, without a pause, by a long and usually louder (stressed) segment that fades gradually towards its termination. This stress (accentuation) of the "articulated" second expiratory segment prepares the patient for the first rhythm of the phonatory exercises proper using vowel play, namely the largo rhythm.

A tone involving vocal fold vibrations is then added to these unvoiced utterances by using the voiced fricative /v/, /z/, and /ʒ/ (Figure 4–8). This step may be used as an intermediate phase prior to the accent exercises coupled with vowel play. It should be stressed that even at this initial preparatory phase of the Accent Method (AM), the therapist-patient interaction is in the form of "a ping-pong" game, in which the patient is trying to copy and (closely) respond to the therapist's performance. This modeling reduces the necessity of explaining the procedure.

Phonatory Phase: Vowel Play

Initially the phonatory exercises take the form of accentuated vowel play. The accentuation (stress) follows specific rhythmic patterns that fit and facilitate the accentuation. These rhythmic exercises are built in a logical hierarchical, manner that helps the patients achieve the final goal of this stage.

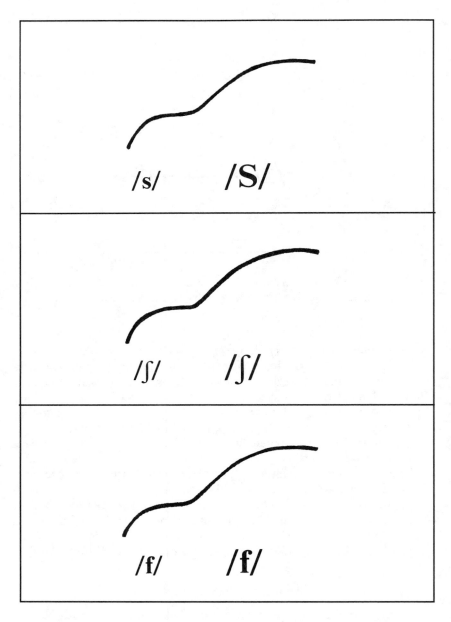

Figure 4–7. An accentuated (crescendo) following the largo tempo utilizing the nonvoiced fricatives /s/ (upper tracing), /ʃ/ (middle tracing) and /f/ (lower tracing). This fricative accentuation prepares the patient for the main part of the accent exercises, namely, vowel play.

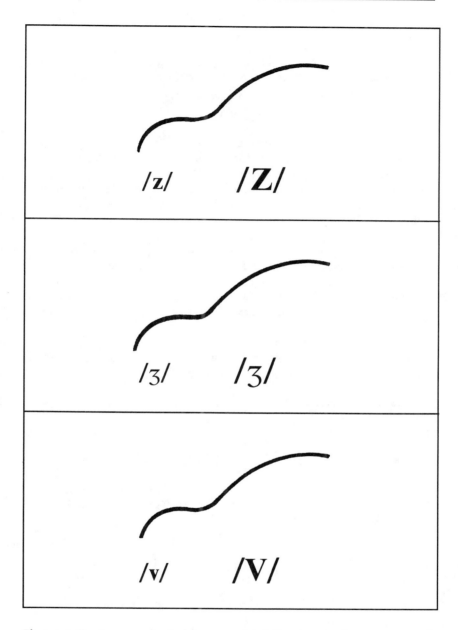

Figure 4–8. An accentuated (crescendo) following the largo tempo utilizing the voiced fricatives /z/ (upper tracing), /ʒ/ (middle tracing), and /v/ (lower tracing).

Largo Rhythm (Tempo I)

Rhythm The first rhythm is a relatively slow one that allows the utterance of a vowel with an initial short, unstressed segment followed by a final long-accentuated segment. This rhythm is a 3/4 beat referred to as largo (Figure 4–9).

Breath Support Breathing is in the form of uninterrupted, cyclic abdomino-diaphragmatic respiration comprising a comfortable inspiration followed by an accentuated expiration. The latter is formed by an initial short-weak segment, followed immediately by a long-accentuated segment. Notice that there is no rest or pause within or between cycles.

Phonatory Exercises This stage of phonatory exercises with vowel play is built logically on the last stage of breathing exercises and the preparatory stage mentioned above. The unstressed/stressed unvoiced, later voiced consonants are turned into a vowel play using the vowel repertoire of the native tongue of the patient. For example:

/a 'a:/, /i 'i:/, /u 'u:/.

The stressed, long /'a:/ terminates by a weak, soft, and unstressed tail.

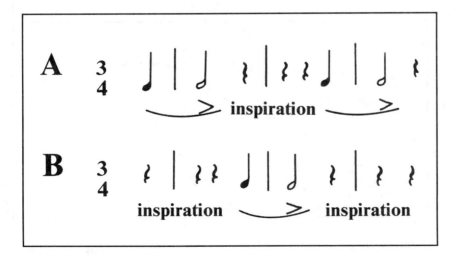

Figure 4–9. The musical notation of the largo rhythm. A, clinician; B, patient.

The goal of the largo rhythm stage of the phonatory accent excersises is to achieve the production of a long, relaxed phonation. To facilitate this goal, the initial stages of this first rhythm are helped by use of a breathy, soft voice. This task may be achieved by asking the patient to attempt an unaccentuated phonation with a lot of initial exhaled air. A short, soft tone is added, to be followed by a tailing stream of air without tone (Figure 4–10). This maneuver thus entails the production of a short soft tone in the middle of an ample expiratory flow. The patient is then advised, while utilizing the largo rhythm to produce an unstressed/ stressed vowel preceded by a short /h/ sound (Figure 4–11). A terminal enhancement of expiratory air flow is observed.

These exercises help to reduce the unwanted initial hard glottal attacks and excessive loudness. The increased final air flow helps to reduce the tendency to vocal fry at the end of the uttered phrases. The patient is gradually led to the production of a tighter and more sonorous voice quality, keeping a final long relaxed phonation.

Associated Body and Arm Movements   To facilitate development of dynamic body movements and the associative activity of voice (later speech production) the patient is guided by the therapist to move the body and limbs while phonating. The type of body move-

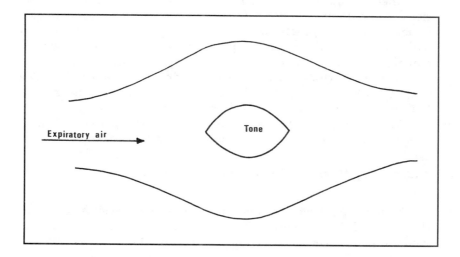

Expiratory air → **Tone**

Figure 4–10. The accent exercises usually start with a breathy voice. There is an ample air flow before, during, and after production of a tone.

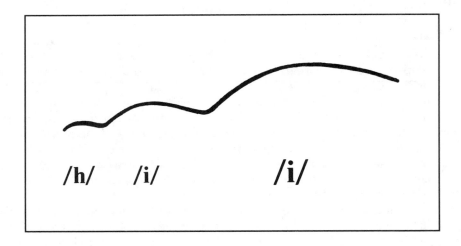

Figure 4–11. The initiation of the accentuated vowel exercises by a /h/ sound helps to reduce the unwanted initial hard glottal attacks and excessive loudness.

ment suitable to the largo rhythm is a forward/backward swaying movement similar to the one introduced with the breathing exercises. The patient, standing on a wide base with one foot forward, is asked to sway gently forward with inspiration and backward with the phonatory expiratory phase while the abdominal wall is moving inward. The back sway starts gently, then increases in magnitude with the vowel accentuation following the largo rhythm. The arms are allowed to sway freely at the side from the shoulder joint. Both movement and sound are fluid.

When the goal of this stage is achieved, the patient is introduced to the second type of rhythmic accentuation of vowel play.

Andante and Allegro Rhythms (Tempo II & III)

Rhythm   At this point, a new rhythm is introduced. It is a faster rhythm, with a 4/4 tempo. The rhythm may have 3 accentuations (andante) or 5 accentuations (allegro) (Figures 4–12 and 4–13).

Breath Support   Before introduction of the andante/allegro tempos, the patient is given an additional instruction in breathing. It is

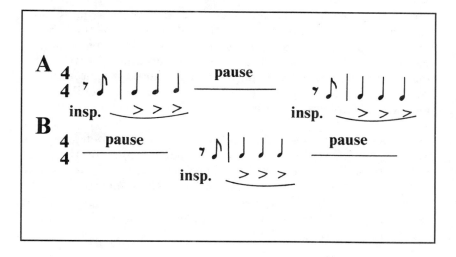

Figure 4–12. The musical notation of the andante rhythm. A, clinician; B, patient.

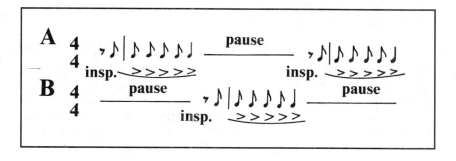

Figure 4–13. The musical notation of the allegro rhythm. A, clinician; B, patient.

indicated to the patient that, in these new tempos, the inspiratory phase (still being abdomino-diaphragmatic), is quick and deep. Inspiration is taken immediately before the vocal utterance. After the vocal utterance the patient is asked to pause in a relaxed manner until his or her turn for vocal utterance in this "ping-pong" game has come. During the pause, the patient's body is relaxed and arms hang freely at his or her side. At the critical moment, just before the vocal utterance, the patient inhales quickly with a deep abdomino-diaphragmatic inspiration in preparation for the following vocal utterance. This breathing maneuver is more similar to the one used in connected speech.

Phonatory Exercises　The goal of this type of vowel play is to transfer the newly acquired smooth relaxed voice of the largo rhythm to production of a series of short successions (3 for andante and 5 for allegro) of vowel phonations while maintaining the relaxed nature of the vocal production. For example, the rhythms practiced are repeated across the exhaled volume of air, thus producing a vowel string like this:

/i 'i:/ for largo

/i 'i'i'i:/, /a 'a'a'a:/ for the andante and

/i 'i'i'i'i'i:/, /a 'a'a'a'a'a:/ for the allegro rhythm,

When a patient finds it difficult to produce a sequence, the individual should return to the initial stages of this phase of phonatory exercises in a soft breathy voice.

Associated Body and Arm Movements　The associative body movements change with the rhythm. With the andante rhythm, movement is in the form of approximately 90° swinging motion around the vertical axis of the body (45° to the right and 45° to the left) to the beat of the rhythm. The upper limbs are allowed to hang freely to follow the body movement. The expressive movements of the arms, however, frequently take the form of rhythmic motions of the forearms at **the elbows**.

With the allegro rhythm, the body movement becomes more of a short, rhythmic, bouncing movement following the relatively fast allegro tempo (Dalhoff & Kitzing, 1987; Smith & Thyme, 1978). Generally there is more vertical motion of the forearms and many expressive movements may be seen with rotation of the hands at the wrists, following the allegro rhythm, much like someone beating a drum with the hands. With practice and change from one rhythm to another, the patient's voice and body movements become increasingly relaxed and free.

When the patient reaches a quasispontaenous stage of using the assocative respiratory-phonatory-articulatory activities, body and arm movements may acquire a more active and varied degree of dramatic expressiveness that suits the articulated vocal utterance (speech).

Stabilization of the Newly Acquired Vocal Behaviors

Attention to Some Phonatory Aspects

At this stage of the therapy program, the new vocal behavior is stabilized by an interplay of the different rhythms (tempos) with accentuated vowel play. The patient is trained also with versatile variations in amplitude (loudness) of the vowel play in order to increase the dynamic range of voice. This part of the program is practiced until the patient masters the production of a **relaxed, sonorous** voice with **variable accentuations** (stresses) and **loudness** while keeping the most suitable and comfortable **pitch**. This aspect constitutes the major sector of the therapy program.

During this phase of the program, the patient is gradually and, as soon as possible, guided to use the newly acquired healthy vocal qualities with the production of nonsense syllables including some consonants. These nonsense syllables will follow the particular prosody of the native tongue of the patient and will bring the newly acquired vocal activities a step closer to connected speech.

Attention to General Posture

During the stage of accentuated vowel play exercises, the clinician indirectly helps the patient **correct faulty postural habits** if those aren't integrated into the natural rhythmic body movements. Exaggerated head extension or neck flexion is corrected by finding the most comfortable position for the patient to "carry" the head, with it being aligned with the rest of the body. High fixed shoulders are eased "down" into a relaxed position.

Attention to the Supralaryngeal Vocal Tract

The clinician encourages the patient to follow his or her example in the production of active movements of the jaw and lips during the vowel play exercises. These movements are usually wide ranged, relaxed, and dynamic. The **activated articulatory movements** help to achieve better projection of the voice/speech message.

The patient is guided to use a **wide pharynx**. The clinician may facilitate this task by referring to the two extremes of accentuated vowel play, one with a tight pharynx and another with a wide pharynx. This is done during the "ping-pong" play of the voice exercises. Phonation with a wide pharynx can be easily demonstrated by phonating while yawning, and phonation with a tight pharynx demonstrated by pulling the tongue back when phonating.

Transfer to Connected Speech

Stages of the Transfer

When the production of the nonsense syllables has been mastered, maintaining the same beneficial healthy voice qualities for all syllable production, the patient is allowed to produce articulated speech in the natural accentuation (stress) of his or her native tongue. Counting and other automatic series (such as recitation of weekdays) are suitable training material for this early stage of articulated phonation. The patient is asked to **repeat** the articulated segments of these series following the manner demonstrated by the clinician. The patient is then asked to repeat parts of selected texts. As soon as this stage is mastered, the patient is introduced to **reading**, applying the same healthy vocal habits to the natural phrasing and prosody of the native tongue (Smith & Thyme 1978). The transfer of the newly acquired vocal habits to connected speech in real-life situations (**monologue** and **dialogue**) is the goal of the final stage of the Accent Method (AM).

Adaptation to the Tempos of the Accent Method

Smith and Thyme (1978) classify the prosodic accentuations (stresses) of connected speech into three language unit/rhythm categories. They suggest that these categories may follow one or the other of the three basic rhythms of the Accent Method (AM) as follows.

Tempo I, Largo   Language units that follow tempo I (largo) may have a conceptual connotation of "isolation." These units usually represent a semantically isolated and outstanding element. To facilitate the patient's awareness of these units while reading, elements belonging to this category are pinpointed in the text by double underlining (=) of the unit concerned.

Examples:

"Good morning,"   "Keep going"

There is one unstressed vowel followed by a stressed (lo-o-o-ong) one.

The movement of the whole arm at the shoulder with the largo rhythm, already practiced at the vowel play phase, may be used at this stage to intensify the feeling of the prosodic accentuations of this category.

Tempo II, Andante Language units that follow tempo II (andante) conceptually have a "selection" connotation. It is used when several items are selected out of a related group or when certain items have to be given equal stress related to a particular concept. Elements belonging to this prosodic category are illustrated in the text used during training of patients by single underlining (_) of the unit concerned.

Examples:

"She is enjoying, charm, beauty, and money"

There is one unstressed vowel followed by 3 stressed (_) vowels.

The movement of the forearm at the elbow, as practiced with the andante vowel play stage, may be used to facilitate this mode of accentuation.

Tempo III, Allegro Language units that follow tempo III (allegro) have a conceptual connotation of "grouping." This is applied when successive semantic units may be grouped for convenience. Elements belonging to this prosodic category are illustrated in the written text by short underlining joined together (⌐____⌐).

Examples:

"I came, you surely remember this."

There are several related stressed vowels in rapid succession, grouped together.

Quick hand movements at the wrist, as practiced with the allegro vowel play phase of the accent exercises, may facilitate the feeling of this type of accentuation while reading.

These exercises are applied to reading, then to monologue, and finally carried into a conversational situation (dialogue). In the early phases of this stage, the usual rhythmic beats may be used simultaneously with the speech utterances to facilitate transferring the vocal behaviors with their accentuations from vowel play to connected speech.

Final Targets

It should be stressed that despite the above mentioned guidelines the clinician has several degrees of freedom in applying and adapting this stage of prosodic reading (later dialogue) to the native tongue used. The clinician should ensure that the patient has acquired a better coordination of **well spaced inspirations, better phrasing (and suitable pauses) with optimal speech rate** (Figure 4–14).

In this connection, it should be underscored that the patient has to be cautioned to **avoid speaking on residual air**.

It is equally important to monitor that the patient is still unconsciously using optimal abdomino-diaphragmatic breathing support during connected speech. All efforts should be directed against lapsing into vocal fry at the end of the phrases. Better breath support may reduce this possible defect.

This stage of treatment is continued until the new habits are automatically and naturally used. It should be stressed that in daily life, patients have enough trouble determining "what" to say, without being distracted by thinking "how" to say it. Clinicians need be mindful of this speaker dilemma. By moving slowly through

---

Transfer to Connected Speech

Despite the general guidelines, the clinician enjoys a degree of freedom. The clinician should ensure, however, that the patient has acquired:

- Better coordination of well-spaced inspirations.
- Better phrasing, with suitable pauses.
- Optimal speech rate.
- Avoidance of speaking on residual air.
- Avoidance of vocal fry at the end of the phrase.
- Perpetuated optimal abdominal breath support.

Figure 4–14. Transfer to connected speech.

each stage and making sure the speech body movements are natural, automatic, and relaxed, clinicians can help avoid this common problem in treatment carryover.

PEDAGOLOGICAL ASPECTS OF THE ACCENT METHOD

General Principles

The guiding pedagological principles in the Accent Method (AM) are:

1. The clinician creates a reassuring atmosphere of collegial friendship with the patient. The clinician should stress and reward the positive vocal behaviors, avoiding pointing out and criticizing defects.
2. The clinician serves as a model, optimizing and idealizing the vocal behavior that is needed to be transferred to the patient.
3. The patient has to concentrate attentively and try to follow the clinician. The interplay between the clinician and the patient is in a form of "ping-pong" game. In this interplay, the patient has a chance to rest, relax, and concentrate while the clinician performs. When the patient's turn comes, he or she can copy what the clinician has been performing. There is a rhythmic alternation between work and rest, acting and watching, giving and taking. It should be pointed out that the clinician, being the model, always takes the initiative in every step of the "ping-pong" game. The clinician is demonstrating the behavior and the patient is following, usually with immediate reward (simply a smile) of the acceptable vocal behavior.
4. In correcting and training the respiratory, phonatory, and articulatory activities, the clinician concentrates on one aspect at a time. It may overwhelm and confuse the patient if several factors are presented to the patient simultaneously. In accent training, clinicians do not swamp their patients.
5. The training program is given in steps of escalating difficulty. These steps should be followed according to the patient's ability to grasp and master each stage. If one step is difficult for the patient to master, the clinician moves back one step and ensures that it is mastered before moving forward. Thus to a large degree the patient determines the pace of treatment.

Facilitation and Logistics

The following arrangements and tools may facilitate achieving the goals of the therapy program.

1. Creation of an atmosphere of friendliness and tranquility in the therapy room with minimal sources of distraction.
2. Reduction of ambient noise in the room and elimination of all sources of external noise.
3. Creation of suitable acoustic treatment of the therapy room to enhance listening conditions. This helps the patient follow the clinician's vocal performance and optimize his or her vocal self-monitoring (auditory feedback).
4. Drum beats are used to intensify the various tempos, thus facilitating the patient's ability to hear and follow rhythms at different stages of the therapy program. In cases in which the drum beats distract a patient, simple forms of timing and rhythm-keeping may be used, such as tapping on the table, hand clapping, or foot stamping. It should be stressed again that, although the Accent Method (AM) is known to be the "drumming method," the use of drum beats to intensify the accent exercises is not essential.
5. The use of recording and playback of the voice with audio and/or video devices helps to demonstrate to the patient certain positive behaviors that need to be reinforced. This may help also to monitor and highlight improvement in the overall vocal performance of a patient. This can be an effective reward to help in reassurance and encouragement to the patient that he or she is progressing.

Format

Pace and Duration of Sessions

The Accent Method (AM) therapy program is generally conducted in individual sessions administered two or three times per week for 20 minutes each session. In a few cases, intensive therapy programs consisting of two sessions per day may be needed; this is particularly well suited for patients who have difficulty getting to therapy because of work or geographical location. These patients may have to temporarily move close to the clinic to get a short, intensive Accent Method (AM) treatment program.

Individual or Group Therapy?

Although the Accent Method (AM) of voice therapy is generally given on individual basis—that is, a clinician one-on-one with a patient—the Accent Method (AM) may be given in the form of group therapy in selected situations. For example, groups may be attempted in the case of a homogenous and relatively well informed group of patients (subjects). Such situations may be suitable for instructing students of logopedics (speech pathology) and phoniatrics in the training of their own voices by an expert clinician in the course of their educational program. It may also work for a group of teachers all suffering from similar vocal misuse patterns.

Face-to-Face Therapy or Homework?

Most of the accent exercises are administered on a face-to-face basis. After the patient has mastered the essentials of the vocal techniques, a recorded tape of the accent exercises may be given for "homework" training.

Economy of Time

Economy of time and, secondarily, expenses, as well as reduction of patient's inconvenience, are central goals in administering the Accent Method (AM) of voice therapy. There is no excessive discussion of principles of the technique and there is no unduly long period of time used to provide vocal hygiene advice. The time used for relaxation, with or without listening to music, is eliminated. The clinician leads the patient step-by-step in the hierarchical structure of the Accent Method (AM) rather swiftly. This reduces the time in therapy and expense.

PSYCHOLOGICAL ASPECTS OF THE ACCENT METHOD (AM)

As in most therapy programs that entail readjustment of behavior, the stages of therapy may be retrospectively described according to identification, motivation, modification, approximation, and stabilization.

Identification

When patients enter therapy, they are usually aware of their complaints. An extra effort, however, is made by the Accent Method

(AM) treating team to help the patient identify the type, nature, and the degree of the vocal pathology. In the stage of identification, the clinician points out the relation between the patient's complaint and the Accent Method (AM). This stage of the Accent Method (AM) is short and informative.

Motivation

During the stage of rapport building, the patient is given an idea about the prognosis and the efficacy of the therapy method to help heighten his or her motivation. The patient's questions requiring clarification about therapy procedures are answered. The clinician also tries to study the practical problems of the patient (transportation, work environment, etc.) that might prevent him or her from regularly attending the therapy program or following through on use of a new, relaxed voice. In particularly protracted programs (as for the therapy of contact granuloma and dysarthrophonia) **repeated counseling** to increase the patient's motivation is usually needed. In shorter programs, motivation may be enhanced through positive changes in voice and reductions in vocal fatigue, with no further counseling from the clinician needed.

Modification

This stage represents the heart of the therapy program: The patient is guided to modifying a faulty vocal behavior to reach a healthy one. This modification, or readjustment, of the vocal behavior is facilitated by the tools described under the section of pedagological considerations. In the Accent Method (AM), positive reassurance and reward are basic tools for reinforcing positive, newly acquired vocal behaviors.

Approximation

After initial successful modification, therapy time is spent in obtaining successive approximations of the patient's behavior to that modeled by the clinician. This is achieved through a wide repertoire of vocal activities and situations as described previously.

Stabilization

The newly acquired healthy vocal behavior is stabilized and transferred as an automatic behavior to connected speech. The accentuated vocal exercises are carried out in the natural prosody of the patient's native tongue. This stage of stabilization and generalization usually is a major portion of the therapy program.

THERAPY TERMINATION

Therapy is terminated when the target is reached and the patient or clinician is satisfied with the voice or when no further progress is likely. A level of vocal function has been stabilized. Termination of voice therapy can be difficult. The relatively long, close interaction between patient and clinician makes it difficult to "wean" the patient from treatment. Guidelines discussed in the following section can help clinicians and patients to make decisions about terminating therapy.

Goals

The final goal of the therapy program is tailored to each patient; some will achieve normal voice and some will not. The ideal goal of "normalization" of vocal function may not always be attainable. Tissue changes, neurological disease, or psychological factors can make this goal impossible.

The clinician should set the treatment target for changes in the vocal function based on the diagnostic characteristics and motivation of each case. The clinician must acknowledge limiting factors and prepare the patient to accept the realistic targets for change. This may aid the patient in maximal performance and directing of his or her efforts and energies toward attainable goals.

Duration

Voice Disorders

The Accent Method (AM) therapy program for functional voice disorders usually takes between 20–25 sessions. With organic voice disorders, such as vocal fold paralysis or vocal fold nodules, the therapy program may be a little bit longer. With other conditions, such as contact granuloma, the therapy program is usually protracted, requiring about 70 sessions. In the latter case, ongoing counseling may be needed to help motivate the patient to complete the therapy program.

Dysarthrophonia

In cases of dysarthria, the Accent Method (AM) therapy program is usually prolonged. Counseling to heighten motivation of both the patient and family should be well integrated in the treatment plan. Improvement is slow and changes are subtle, with motivational counseling frequently needed. The general health of a patient may contribute to the problem; the patient may be depressed or unable to attend therapy regularly. Moreover, the goal with some persons with dysarthria may be to maintain voice at a particular level, rather than to achieve normal function. The clinician works for treatment to prevent further deterioration.

Termination Criteria

Guidelines for termination of a therapy program are provided. It should be underscored that these criteria need to be viewed within the previously set goals of therapy for each patient according to his or her condition and potentials. These guidelines fall into four categories:

A. Patient's satisfaction in real-life situations in which he or she employs vocal activities. This means the disappearance (reduction) of a subjective complaint.

B. Improvement and stabilization of the auditory perceptual assessment (APA) of the patient's voice as judged by an experienced clinician. Voice recording is a helpful tool for documenting change.

C. Improvement of the laryngoscopic picture in indirect-micro-laryngo-videostroboscopy or other alternative tools as judged by the phoniatrician or the laryngologist with experience in voice disorders. Documentation is important to ensure targets are reached.

D. Maximal improvement of the patient's phonatory function, as monitored by whatever instrumental measures are available (see Protocol of Assessment—Appendix 1).

Ideally, when the clinician and the phoniatrician (or laryngologist) decide it is time to terminate the therapy program, all four termination parameters have reached target levels. Persistence of a laryngeal pathology or a deviant aspect of vocal function should raise suspicion that there is something wrong with the treatment program or the patient's ability to respond to treatment. The reason for the failure to respond should be determined before treatment is terminated.

Factors Influencing Prognosis

The main factor determining the success of the Accent Method (AM) is the **proper choice of patients**. Faulty choice of patients or indiscriminate application of the Accent Method (AM) may lead to unjustified disappointments. The skill level, education, and experience of the clinician are also important factors contributing to the success or failure of the therapy program.

There are also factors related to the patient that may influence prognosis. Musicality (Bergendal, 1976) and high motivation are positive prognostic factors, with hearing impairment possibly presenting an obstacle to the therapy program.

The rate of relapses (recurrence of symptoms), estimated from clinical populations returning for treatment, is low. The successful readjustment of the general health habits and vocal behaviors to avoid further injury is the central key to reduction of relapses.

THERAPEUTIC EFFICACY

Few studies have objectively tackled the question of efficacy of voice therapy. The therapeutic efficacy of the Accent Method (AM), although known for decades to be clinically effective across many cultures and languages, has only recently been investigated. The last two decades of research, though somewhat sparse, have demonstrated its effectiveness as measured by change in acoustic, electroglottography (EGG), and aerodynamic recordings.

Smith and Thyme (1976) studied the effect of a short-term therapy course (10 sessions) on the voice of 30 students of a teachers' college. The reseachers utilized an acoustic analysis battery. The posttherapy measurements showed an increased intensity across the whole frequency spectrum, particularly below 1000 Hz. The researchers concluded that the Accent Method (AM) was efficacious and that the increased energy below 1000 Hz may be responsible for the improvement in speech intelligibility and in giving the impression of a fuller voice.

Thyme and Frökjaer-Jensen (1983) presented the results of a short intensive voice therapy program (4 hours daily for 5 days) given to 16 trained speech pathologists (logopedists). Instrumental assessment of voice was based on electroglottography (EGG) and phonetographic (Voice Range Profile-[VRP]) recordings made pre- and posttreatment. EGG showed a longer glottal closure. The phonetograms (VRP) showed an increase in the "phonatory area" (or voice field) by a total of 3.3 semitones. The upper notes were increased by 1.7 semitones, and the lower ones were lowered by 1.6 semitones. The maximum dynamic range was increased by 10.6 dB.

Frökjaer-Jensen and Prytz (1976) studied the effect of the accent exercises on long time average spectral analysis (LTAS) of the patient's voice. They found that the main beneficial change in response to therapy was an increase in the energy in the frequency range above 1000 Hz. This was thought to reflect the clearer timbre (quality) of voice.

Löfqvist (1986) found a tendency of the accent exercises to increase the ratio of LTAS energy above 1000 Hz relative to the energy below 1000 Hz. He recommended use of this acoustic tool to study intraperson changes rather than interperson changes.

Kotby, El-Sady, Bassiouny, Abou-Rass, and Hegazi (1991) studied the efficacy of the Accent Method (AM) in treating several categories of voice disorders. Three main etiological groups were studied, namely: nonorganic (functional) voice disorders, nodules, and vocal fold paralysis with persistent glottal gap. The study was carried out on 28 patients. The diagnostic workup provided information in four areas:

1. Patient's own evaluation of the change in the degree of the symptoms.
2. Auditory perceptual assessment (APA) as judged by experienced clinicians following a modified GRBAS scale (Hirano, 1981).
3. Visual assessment and documentation utilizing indirect-micro-laryngo-videostroboscopy, with measurements of the changes in size of the lesion (nodule or glottal gap).
4. Aerodynamic studies measuring several parameters (Table 4–1).

Reevaluation using the same assessment battery was done after 10 sessions and again after 20 sessions of voice therapy. The patients' self-analysis showed a positive grade shift in 25 out of 28 subjects. The number of grade shifts varied. The improvement in APA showed a positive grade shift in the overall grade in 19 cases. The strained voice quality showed a positive grade shift in 14 cases, whereas the leaky quality showed positive grade shift in 12 cases. The breathy and the irregular qualities did not show significant positive shifts.

Changes in the measurements of the organic lesion (nodule and glottal gap) from indirect-micro-laryngo-videostroboscopy were observed as a reduction of size of the nodule in all 6 cases (Figure 4–15) and a reduction of the glottal gap in 4 cases out of 6 (Figures 4–16 and 4–17). In two cases of vocal fold paralysis with glottal gap, the gap disappeared completely.

Aerodynamic parameters showed significant improvement in maximum phonation time (MPT), mean flow rate (MFR), subglottal pressure (Psub), and glottal efficiency (GE), with vital capacity

Table 4–1. Ranges of aerodynamic parameters for normal speakers across age and gender differences.

Parameters	Ranges	Authors
Vital capacity (in ml)	1280–4530	Kotby et al., 1990
Maximum phonation time (in seconds)	15–35 3.8–36.3	Hirano, 1981 Kotby et al., 1990
Phonatory quotient	120–160 60–447	Hirano, 1981 Kotby et al., 1990
Mean flow rate (in ml/sec)	40–200 52–178	Hirano, 1981 Kotby et al., 1990
Subglottal pressure (in cm H_2O)	3.5–50 2–35 6.4–22.2	Van den Berg, 1955 Schutte, 1992 Kotby et al., 1990
Glottal resistance in cm H_2O/L/sec)	30–40 12–93 46–145	Smitheran & Hixon, 1981 Holmberg et al., 1988 Kotby et al., 1990

Glottal efficiency [x E-05]
  at 40 dB
  at normal loudness
  at 47 db
  at normal loudness
	
	0.45–45
	0.35–145.2
	0.12–400
	20–200
		
		Van den Berg, 1955
		Holmberg et al., 1988
		Schutte, 1992
		Kotby et al., 1990

(VC), phonatory quotient (PQ), and glottal resistance (GR) not showing a significant positive change (Table 4–2).

Kotby et al. (1991) conclude that the Accent Method (AM) is therapeutically effective in nonorganic (functional) voice disorders, vocal nodules, and paralysis of vocal folds. They recommend that the Accent Method (AM), may be indicated as the treatment of choice in cases of soft nodules with a base of < 2.5 mm and an elevation (rise) of < 0.5 mm. They also show that patients with a glottal gap of 1 mm or less responded positively to Accent Method (AM) voice therapy, alone. Larger gaps may need preliminary surgical intervention before the initiation of accent voice exercises. They endorse accent exercises postoperatively as a supplementary line of treatment to optimize the voice results.

Although not included in the study, Kotby et al. (1991) find that contact granuloma also responds positively to the Accent Method (AM) voice therapy (Figure 4–18).

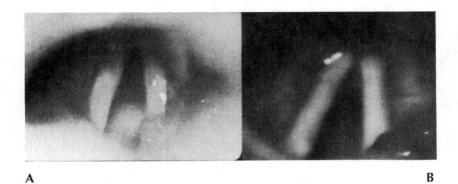

A   B

Figure 4–15. Bilateral vocal fold nodules. A: before therapy, B. after therapy.

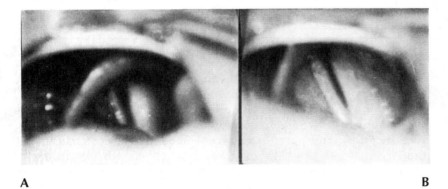

A   B

Figure 4–16. Right vocal fold paralysis with a glottic gap seen in ordinary light. A: before therapy, B: after therapy.

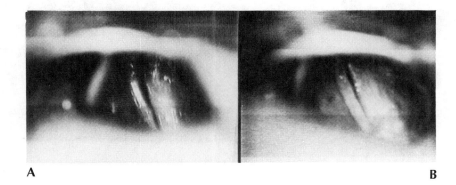

A   B

Figure 4–17. Right vocal fold paralysis with a glottic gap seen in stroboscopic light. A: before therapy, B. after therapy.

Table 4–2. Aerodynamic results for 28 voice-disordered patients before and after Accent Method voice therapy

	Mean Value		Paired "t" Test Values	
	Before	**After**		
VC (ml)	2750	2690	t = 0.88	P>0.05, NS
MPT (sec)	10.1	12.0	t = 2.20	P<0.05, SIG
PQ	403	314	t = 1.80	P>0.05, NS
MFR (ml/s)	282	216	t = 2.76	P<0.01, SIG
Psub (cm H$_2$O)	114	99	t = 3.00	P<0.01, SIG
GE (X E-05)	3.8	5.8	t = 2.68	P<0.05, SIG
GR (cm H$_2$O/L/s)	0.521	0.643	t = 1.57	P>0.05, NS

MPT = maximum phonation time; PQ = phonatory quotient; MFR = mean flow rate; Psub = subglottal pressure; GE = glottal efficiency; GR = glottal resistance; SIG = significant; NS = Non-significant.

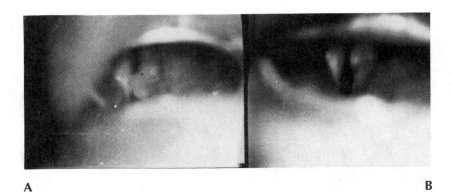

A   B

Figure 4–18. Left vocal fold contact granuloma. A: before therapy, B: after therapy.

Fex, Fex, Shiromoto, and Hirano (1994) evaluated the efficacy of the Accent Method (AM) as determined from acoustic measures made pre- and posttreatment. Ten patients with functional dysphonia were reevaluated after 10 therapy sessions. The authors find that the parameters of pitch perturbation quotient (PPQ), normalized noise energy (NNEa), and F_0 changed toward normalization after therapy by the Accent Method (AM).

CLOSING REMARKS

The Accent Method (AM) may be considered an exotic voice therapy method by clinicians unfamiliar with the techniques, because the rhythms and body movements integral to the technique make some clinicians uncomfortable. It is this rhythmic activity that may help make therapy more fluid for both the clinician and the patient. Nevertheless, it should be stressed that drum beat enhancement of the accentuated rhythm in the Accent Method (AM) is not an essential prerequisite for carrying out the accent exercises.

The Accent Method (AM), although highly structured, need not be conducted with an authoritarian attitude. During the behavior readjustment therapy program, it is important to respect and preserve the personal voice and speech traits (identities) of each patient. The patient should be helped to sound better, but like himself or herself, not like cookie cutter voices or talking robots.

Improved phonatory articulatory behavior is more easily achieved when it occurs without the patient's awareness. "Awareness" often leads to unnecessary and unavoidable tension. The therapist should not be preoccupied by the trainee's faults, but by what the trainee is able to produce correctly. The clinician should constantly "visualize" the state of the vocal tract while acoustically monitoring the vocal outcome. The clinician should keep the diagnostic data profile of the patient in mind while guiding him or her to vocal safety and improved vocal function. Fundamental to change is a realistic scientifically based image of the pathophysiology underlying a disorder. The "battle" of vocal behavior readjustment is made easier and more effective when led by a multidisciplinary team of speech pathologists (logopedists), phoniatricians, and laryngologists working in close cooperation. In some instances, vocal coaches and counselors are also part of the team.

The Accent Method (AM) is a good instrument. It awaits, however, the well-trained clinician to "play" it well to achieve optimal use of its potentials to modify vocal behavior.

The Accent Method (AM) is probably not unique from the pure technical point of view. Breathing, rhythm, and coordinated dynamic phonatory/articulatory movements have been described by various other methods of voice therapy (Forchhammer, 1974; Froeschels, 1952; Sovijarvi, 1984). Smith's unique contribution is that he presented his Accent Method (AM) as a logically built and holistically based stepwise technique. Moreover, he attempted to provide a rationale for the Accent Method (AM) that has helped to transfer it from a pure art treatment to a systematic practice more closely aligned with science.

REFERENCES

Bergendal, B. I. (1976). Musical talent testing used as a prognostic instrument in voice treatment. *Folia Phoniatrica* (Basel), *28*, 8.

Boone, D. R. (1988). *The voice and voice therapy* (4th ed.). Englewood Cliffs, NJ: Prentice-Hall.

Dalhoff, K., & Kitzing, P. (1987). Voice therapy according to Smith comments on the Accent Method to treat disorders of voice and speech. *Journal of Research in Singing and Applied Vocal Pedagogy, 11*(1), 15.

Fex, B., Fex, S., Shiromoto, O., & Hirano, M. (1994). Acoustic analysis of functional dysphonia: Before and after voice therapy (Accent Method). *Journal of Voice, 8*(2), 163.

Forchhammer, E. (1974). *Stemmens Funktioner Og fejlfunktioner*. Copenhagen, Denmark: Munksgaard.

Froeschels, E. (1952). Chewing method as therapy: A discussion with some philosophical conclusions. *Archives of Otolaryngology, 56*, 427.

Frökjaer-Jensen, B., & Prytz, S. (1976). Registration of voice quality. *Brüel & Kjaer Technical Review, 3*, 3–17.

Greene, M. C. L. (1980). *The voice and its disorders* (4th ed.). Philadelphia: J. B. Lippincott Company.

Hirano, M. (1981). *Clinical examination of voice*. New York: Springer-Verlag.

Holmberg, E. B., Hillman, R. E., & Perkell, J. S. (1988). Glottal air flow and transglottal air pressure measurements for male and female speakers in soft, normal and loud voice. *The Journal of the Acoustical Society of America, 84*(2), 511.

Kotby, M. N., Barakah, M.S., Abou El-Ella, M.Y., Khidre, A.A., & Hegazi, M.A. (1990). Aerodynamic analysis of voice disorders. In T. Sacristàn, J. J. Alvarez-Vicent, J. Bartual, F. Antoli-Candela, & L.Rubio (Eds.), *Otorhinolaryngology, Head & Neck Surgery. Proceedings of the XIV Congress of Otorhinolaryngology, Head and Neck Surgery* (Vol. II) (p. 2041). Amsterdam: Kugler and Ghedini Publication.

Kotby, M. N., El-Sady, S. R., Bassiouny, S. E., Abou-Rass, Y. A., & Hegazi, M. A. (1991). Efficacy of the Accent Method of voice therapy. *Journal of Voice, 5*(4), 316.

Lauritzen, K. (1970). Om Taleundervisning efter accentmetoden. *Medlems-blad fur Talepaedagogisk Forening, 132*.

Löfqvist, A. (1986). Long-time-average spectrum as a tool in voice research. *Journal of Phonetics, 14*, 471.

Luchsinger, R., & Arnold, G. E. (1965). *Voice-speech-language*. Belmont, CA: Wadsworth Publishing Company, Inc.

Schutte, H. K. (1992). Integrated aerodynamic measurements. *Journal of Voice, 6*(2), 127.

Smitheran, J. R., & Hixon, T. J. (1981). A clinical method for estimating laryngeal airway resistance during vowel production. *Journal of Speech and Hearing Disorders, 46*, 138.

Smith, S., & Thyme, K. (1976). Statistic research on changes in speech due to pedagogic treatment (the Accent Method). *Folia Phoniatrica* (Basel), *28*, 98.

Smith, S., & Thyme, K. (1978). *Accentmetoden*. Herning, Denmark: Special Paedagogisk Forlag.

Sovijarvi, A. (1984). Some therapeutic exercises for rehabilitating functional dysphonias presented on videotape. In *The study of sounds. The Proceedings of the Fourth World Congress of Phoneticians* (Vol. XX) (pp. 445–457). Japan: The Phonetic Society of Japan.

Thyme, K., & Frökjaer-Jensen, B. (1983). Results of one week's intensive voice therapy (the Accent Method). *Proceedings of the XIX International Association of Logopedics and Phoniatrics Congress 894*. Edinburgh, Scotland.

Van den Berg, J. W. (1955). Direct and indirect determination of the mean subglottic pressure. *Folia Phoniatrica* (Basel), *8*, 1.

APPENDIX 1

PROTOCOL FOR VOICE EVALUATION

Serial no.:   Date:

I. ELEMENTARY DIAGNOSTIC PROCEDURES:

These are possible to apply in primary care voice clinics. It needs simple hardware.

(A) Patient Interview:

(1) *Personal Data:*

Name: DOB: Sex:
Residence:
Marital status: Number of children: Age(s):
Education:
Occupation:

(2) *Complaint and Analysis of Symptoms:*

-
-
- Duration
- Onset: gradual
        sudden   following   __acute major voice abuse
                                    __acute upper respiratory tract
                                      infection
                                    __no detectable reason
- Course: stable   increasing   intermittent   decreasing
- Phonasthenic symptoms (vocal fatigue):
    __Throat dryness/soreness
    __Throat tenderness
    __Frequent throat clearing
    __Difficulty in swallowing sticky throat mucus (Globus!)

(3) *Impact of Complaint on the Patient:*

- Patient's self-rating of the severity:

0	1	2	3	4

  (no effect)   (severe handicap)
- Effect on daily life:
- Listener's reaction (patient's viewpoint):

(4) *Search for Etiological Factors:*

- Type of Job:
  - Vocal demand: high   moderate   low
  - Number of hours of exposure to vocal demand per day:
- Job Environment:
  - Level of ambient noise:
  - Reverberation time:
  - Relative humidity:
  - Temperature:
  - Irritants: dust   amount   particle size
                      fumes   type   concentration
- Smoking: quantity   duration   past history
- Alcohol use: quantity   duration   past history
- Temperament: quiet   tense
- Emotional stress:
- Repeated U.R.T. infection: frequency
- Allergic tendencies:
- Rheumatic/rheumatoid symptoms:
- Chronic cough and chest diseases:
- Breathing: dyspnea
- Chewing & swallowing:
- Hyperacidity & reflux:
- Medications:
- Surgical interventions & trauma:

(5) *Factors that Might Influence Therapy:*

- Hearing: • Musicality:

(B) Auditory Perceptual Assesment (APA) (Hirano, 1981; Kotby, 1986)

	(0) normal	(1) slight	(2) moderate	(3) severe

- Overall grade:
- Character (quality):
  - Strained (S)
  - Leaky (L)
  - Breathy (B)
  - Irregular (Rough) (I)
- Pitch:
  - Overall increase   decrease
  - Diplophonia
- Register:
  - Habitual register: modal   falsetto
  - Tendency of vocal fry at the end of phrase
  - Register break
- Loudness:
  - Excessively loud   excessively soft
  - Fluctuating
- Glottal attack: normal   soft   hard
- Associated laryngeal functions: cough   whisper   laughter
- Tape recording: No.:

(C) E.N.T. Examination
- Oral Cavity:
- Pharynx: Tonsils   post-nasal discharge
- Nasal Cavity:
- Ears:

(D) Type of Breathing: __ Upper costal   __ Diaphragmatic

(E) Head Position: __ Normal   __ Overflexed
__ Overextended   __ Other

(F) Laryngeal Examination:

1. *External Laryngeal Examination:*

- Laryngeal skeleton:
    Normal configuration
    Fractures: site   type
    Other abnormalities
- Laryngeal click: normal   absent
- Laryngeal position: high   normal   low
- Cervical veins: normal   engorged
- Neck scars: Type   site   dimensions

2. *Elementary Visual Impression and Mirror Laryngoscopy:*
   (Garcia, 1855)

(i) Structures to be examined: (see diagram)

1. Vallecula
2. Epiglottis
3. Aryepiglottic
   folds
4. Vocal folds
5. Anterior
   commissure

6. Subglottis
7. Ventricular bands
8. Ventricles
9. Arytenoids
10. Interarytenoid
11. Postcricoid region
12. Pyriform fossae

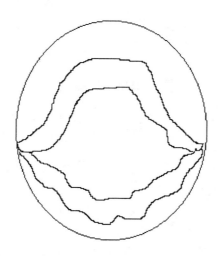

(ii) Items to be noticed:

1. Mucous membrane
2. Vocal folds configuration:
3. Vocal folds movements:
   - Gross movements:
   - Phonatory coaptation (phonatory vocal fold closure):
4. Ventricular folds:

II. CLINICAL DIAGNOSTIC AIDS:

These are possible to apply in specialized voice clinics. The procedures are feasible and are essentially noninvasive.

1. Augmentation & Documentation of the Glottic Picture:

- Indirect microlaryngoscopy (Seidner et al., 1972)
- Telescopic rigid fiber orolaryngoscopy (Yoshida & Hirano, 1979)
- Flexible nasofibrolaryngoscopy (Sataloff et al., 1990; Sawashima & Ushijima, 1971).

A. Continuous light

(I) Vocal Folds:
(a) Mucous Membrane:

–Color:	Pale	red	white	others
–Luster:	wet	dry		
–Transparency:	shiny		opaque	
–Vascular markings:	few	many	hematoma	
–Swelling	site	size	shape	
	edge	surface	color	
–Ulcers	site	size	floor	edge
–Girth	normal	hypertrophy	atrophy	

(b) Configurations:
   –Symmetry of the glottis
   –Deviation of the glottis   direction   degree
(c) Movements
   –Gross mobility: (Adduction/abduction)
          Restricted   right   left
          Fixed   right   left
          Glottic gap (size posteriorly in mm.)
   –Phonatory coaptation (phonatory vocal fold closure):
          normal:

gap: size (posteriorly in mm)   site
change on more active phonation
(II) Ventricular Folds:
   –Mucous membrane: color   masses
   –Girth   normal   hypertrophy   atrophy
   –Position at phonation   normal   adducted

B. Stroboscopy: (Hirano & Bless, 1993; Saito et al., 1978; Schönhärl, 1960; Timcke, von Leden, & Moore, 1959; Wendler, 1977; Winckel, 1965)

(i) Phonatory test characteristics:
   –Fundamental frequency:
   –Intensity:
(ii) Configuration:
   –Glottic closure: complete   incomplete
   –Glottic gap: site   size
   –Amplitude: great   normal   small   zero
    RT.
    LT.
   –Glottic wave: great   normal   small   absent
    RT.
    LT.
   –Symmetry: in phase   in amplitude
   –Phase closure: open phase predominate
                  closed phase predominate
   –Stroboscopic fixation: segment   side
   –Additional morphological findings and details:

Documentation and measurement: (Fex et al., 1991; Hibi et al., 1988; Peppard & Bless, 1990; Sercarz et al., 1991)

- Videostroboscopy
- Video-printouts

2. Voice Recording:

- Sound treated room   • Apparatus
   –Microphone distance
   –Material
     • standardized text
     • counting
     • sustained vowel phonation   /a/   /i/   /u/

III. ADDITIONAL INSTRUMENTAL DIAGNOSTIC MEASURES:

These are fit for application in highly specialized voice laboratories. The hardware, although noninvasive, is expensive and requires a high degree of competence to operate.

(1) **Acoustic Analysis:** (Davis, 1981; Hirano, 1989; Ludlow et al., 1985; Saleh, 1991)

- Fundamental frequency (F_0)
- Long time average spectral analysis (LTAS) (Frökjaer-Jensen & Prytz, 1976)
- Perturbation of frequency (Jitter) (Baken & Daniloff, 1991; Milenkovic, 1987)
- Perturbation of amplitude (Shimmer)
- Relative energy level (as signal to noise ratio)

(2) **Aerodynamic Measures:** (Hirano, 1989; Kotby et al, 1990; Rothenberg, 1973; Schutte, 1992; Tanaka & Gould, 1985; Yanagihara, 1969)

Elementary measures:

- Vital capacity (VC)
- Maximum phonation time (MPT)
- Phonatory quotient (PQ) = VC/MPT

Additional measures and indices:

- Fundamental frequency (F_0):   habitual   range
- Sound pressure level (SPL)   habitual   range
- Mean flow rate (MFR in ml/sec)
- Subglottic pressure (Psub in cm H_2O)
- Glottis-vocal tract system efficiency
  (GVTE) = I / Psub $\times$ MFR
- Glottal resistance (GR in cm H_2O/L/sec) = Psub/MFR

(3) **Voice Range Profile (Phonetogram):** Damsté, 1970; Gramming, 1988; Hacki, 1988)

	Extent	Distribution	Area
Speaking voice			
Shouting voice			
Singing voice			

(4) **Radiological Studies:**

- Plain X-ray
- CT scanning (Mancuso & Hanafee, 1988)
- Magnetic resonance imaging (MRI) (Lufkin & Hanafee, 1989)
- Laryngo-pharyngo-esophageal videofluoroscopy

(5) **Electromyography (EMG)**: (Dejonckere, 1987; Hirano & Ohala, 1969; Kotby & Haugen, 1970; Kotby et al., 1992; Thumfart, 1988)

Inferior Laryngeal nerve (ILN)—Thyroarytenoid muscle
Superior Laryngeal nerve (SLN)—Cricothyroid muscle
- Electrical silence:
- Spontaneous activity
          fibrillation   positive denervation potential
- Interference pattern: full   incomplete
- Mean duration and amplitude of MUAP: (Histogram)
- Symmetry of the changes:

(6) **Glottography (EGG)/(PGG):** (Fourcin, 1974; Kelman, 1981; Kitzing, 1979; Lecluse, 1974)

- Non-acoustic measures of F_3
- Glottic area waveform (vocal fold contact area) (Baken, 1987)
- Open quotient (OQ) = Open phase/entire phase
- Speed quotient (SQ)= Opening phase/closing phase
- Speed index (SI) = SQ $-$ 1 / SQ + 1
- Onset/offset characteristics

REFERENCES

Baken, R. J. (1987). *Clinical measurement of speech and voice.* Boston: College-Hill Press.

Baken, R. J., & Daniloff, R. G. (1991). *Readings in clinical spectrography of speech.* San Diego: Singular Publishing Group.

Damsté, P. H. (1970). The phonetogram. *Practica Oto-Rhino-Laryngologica, 32,* 185.

Davis, S. B. (1981). Acoustic characteristics of normal and pathological voices. Proceedings of the conference on the assessment of vocal pathology. *ASHA Reports, 11,* 97.

Dejonckere, P. H. (1987). *E.M.G. of the larynx.* Louvain, Belgium: Marc Pietteur.

Fex, S., Fex, B.,& Hirano, M. (1991). A clinical procedure for linear measurements at the vocal fold level. *Journal of Voice, 5,* 328.

Fourcin, A. J. (1974). Laryngographic examination of vocal fold vibration. In B. Wyke (Ed.), *Ventilatory and phonatory control systems,* (p. 315). London: Oxford University Press.

Frökjaer-Jensen, B., & Prytz, S. (1976). Registration of voice quality. *Brüel and Kjaer Technical Review, 3,* 3–17

Garcia, M. (1885). Physiological observations on the human voice. *Proceedings Royal Society,* London, 399.

Gramming, P. (1988). *The phonetogram. An experimental and clinical study.* Malmö, Sweden: Lidbergs Blankett AB.

Hacki, T. (1988). Evaluation of the quantitative speaking voice production: The phonetogram of the speaking voice in relation to that of the singing voice. *Folia Phoniatrica* (Basel), *40,* 190.

Hibi, S. R., Bless, D. M., Hirano, M. ,& Yoshida, T. (1988). Distortions of videofiberoscopy imaging: Reconsideration and correction. *Journal of Voice, 2,* 168.

Hirano, M. (1981). *Clinical examination of voice.* New York: Springer-Verlag.

Hirano, M. (1989). Objective evaluation of human voice. Clinical aspects. *Folia Phoniatrica* (Basel), *41,* 89.

Hirano, M., & Ohala, J. (1969). Use of hooked-wire electrodes for electromyography of the intrinsic laryngeal muscles. *Journal of Speech and Hearing Research, 12,* 362.

Kelman, A. W. (1981). Vibratory pattern of the vocal folds. *Folia Phoniatrica* (Basel), *33,* 73.

Kitzing, P. (1979). *Glottografisk Frekvensindikering.* Malmo: MAS Tryckeri/Litos Reprotryck i Malmö AB.

Kotby, M. N. (1986). Voice disorders: Recent diagnostic advances. *Egyptian Journal of Otolaryngology, 3*(1), 69.

Kotby, M. N, Barakah, M. A., Abou El-Ella, M. Y., Khidr A. A., & Hegazi M. A. (1990). Aerodynamic analysis of voice disorders. In T. Sacristán, J. J. Alvarez-Vicent, J. Bartual, F. Antoli-Candela, & L. Rubio (Eds.), Otorhinolaryngology, Head and Neck Surgery. *Proceedings of XIV World Congress of Otorhinolaryngology, Head and Neck Surgery* (Vol II) (p. 2041). Amsterdam: Kugler and Ghedini Publication.

Kotby, M. N., Fadly, E., Madkour, O., Barakah, M., Khidr, A., Alloush, T., & Saleh, H. (1992). Electromyography and neurography in neurolaryngology. *Journal of Voice, 6*(2), 159.

Kotby, M. N., & Haugen, L. K. (1970). Clinical appplication of electromyography in vocal fold mobility disorders. *Acta Otolaryngologica (Stockholm), 70,* 428.

Lecluse, F. L. E. (1974). Laboratory investigations in electroglottography. *Proceedings of the 16th International Congress of Logopedics and Phoniatrics, Interlaken,* Switzerland, 294.

Ludlow, C. L., Bassich, C. J., Connor, N. P., Coulter, D. C., & Lee, Y. J. (1985). The validity of using phonatory jitter and shimmer to detect laryngeal pathology. In C. Sasaki, K. Harris, & T. Baer (Eds.), *Vocal fold physiology: Laryngeal function in phonation and respiration* (Vol.VIII) (p. 492). Boston: College-Hill Press.

Lufkin, R. B., Larsson, S. G., & Hanafee, W. N. (1983). Work in progress: NMR of the larynx and tongue base. *Radiology, 148,* 173.

Mancuso, A. A., & Hanafee W. N. (1982). *Computed tomography of the head and neck.* Baltimore: Williams and Wilkins.

Milenkovic, P. (1987). Least mean square measurement of voice perturbation, *Journal of Speech and Hearing Research, 30,* 529.

Peppard, R. D., & Bless, D. M. (1990). A method for improving measurement reliability in laryngeal video-stroboscopy. *Journal of Voice, 4,* 280.

Rothenberg, M. (1973). A new inverse filtering technique for deriving the glottal wave form during voicing. *Journal of Acoustic Society of America, 53,* 1623.

Saito, S., Fukuda, H., Kitahara, S., & Kokawa, N. (1978). Stroboscopic observation of vocal fold vibration with fiberoptics. *Folia Phoniatrica* (Basel), *30,* 241.

Saleh, M. S. (1991). *Acoustic analysis of voice in certain types of dysphonia.* Unpublished doctoral dissertation, Department of Phoniatrics, Faculty of Medicine, Ain Shams University, Cairo.

Sataloff, R. T., Spiegel, J. R., Carroll, L. M., Darby, K. S., Hawkshaw, M. J.,& Rulnick, R. (1990). The clinical voice laboratory: Practical design and clinical application. *Journal of Voice, 4,* 264.

Sawashima, M., & Ushijima, T. (1971). Use of fiberscope in speech research. *Annual Bulletin, Research Institute of Logopedics and Phoniatrics (No. 5).* University of Tokyo, 25.

Schönhärl, E. (1960). *Die stroboskopie in Der Praktischen Laryngologie.* Stuttgart: George Thieme Verlag.

Schutte, H. K. (1992). Integrated aerodynamic measurements. *Journal of Voice,* 6(2), 127.

Seidner, W., Wendler, J., & Malbedi, G. (1972). Mikrostroboscopie. *Folia Phoniatrica* (Basel), *24,* 81.

Sercarz, J. A., Berke, G. S., Arnstein, D., Gerratt, B., & Natividad, M. (1991). A new technique for quantitative measurement of laryngeal videostroscopic images. *Archives of Otolaryngology, Head and Neck Surgery, 117,* 871.

Tanaka, S., & Gould, W. J. (1985). Vocal efficiency and aerodynamic aspects in voice disorders. *Annals of Otology, Rhinology & Laryngology, 94,* 29.

Thumfart, W. F. (1988). From larynx to vocal ability. New electrophysiological data. *Acta Otolaryngologica (Stockholm), 105,* 425.

Timcke, R., von Leden, H., & Moore, P. (1959). Laryngeal vibrations: Measurements of the glottic wave. Part II: Physiologic variations. *Archives of Otolaryngology, 69,* 438.

Wendler, J. (1977). *Practical hints for the application of laryngo-stroboscopy.* Dresden: VEB Trasformatoren-und Rontgenwerk "Hermann Matern."

Winckel, F. (1965). Phoniatric acoustics. In R.L. Luchsinger, & G. E. Arnold (Eds.), *Voice-speech-language* (pp. 24–55) Belmont, CA: Wadsworth Publishing Company, Inc.

Yoshida, Y., & Hirano, M. (1979). A video-tape recording system for laryngeal stroboscopy. *Journal of Japan Bronchoesophagological Society, 30,* 1.

APPENDIX 2

I. SOVIJARVI'S STABILIZATION EXERCISES FOR VOICE THERAPY

Sovijarvi (1974) noticed the presence of faulty postures of the laryngeal cartilages and/or the hyoid bone in a great number of his patients (75.3%). These defective postures included:

(1) Inclination or twisting of the thyroid cartilage to one side.
(2) Twisting and/or elevation of the hyoid bone.
(3) Twisting of the cricoid cartilage.

Sovijarvi believes that these faulty postures are mostly acquired by habitual faulty positions during work, sleep, or speaking on the phone and are more common in men than women. He claims that these postural asymmetries play an important role in the pathogenesis of nonorganic (functional) voice disorders, particularly of the larynx as related to defective control of pitch and loudness. The functional imbalances arise when the inclination or twisting reaches 2–3 mm.

Sovijarvi (1984) has introduced what he called the "Stabilization Phenomenon" Method to achieve functional balance (synergism) of the extrinsic laryngeal musculature and correct laryngeal frame asymmetries. This method achieves a synchronous lowering of the whole laryngeal frame (interior stabilization) and the elastic forward downward motion of the hyoid bone (superior stabilization).

The program begins with a thorough palpation of the patient's laryngeal region; physical findings from this palpation serve as the bases for the "stabilization" exercise program.

Sovijarvi's method of diverse related specific exercises incorporates specific exercises for different treatment phases. The preparatory phase of breathing exercises stresses the importance of the lower thoracic (abdominal) deep breathing. Sovijarvi has developed his phonatory drills by drawing from his vast experience as a phonetician. He describes certain logatomes (nonsense words) having a special phonetic structure with several specified consonant/vowel combinations. These logatomes are designed to correct specific postural defects of the hyoid bone and laryngeal cartilages. This goal is thought to be assisted by certain body movements (e.g. disc throwing). Sovijarvi claims that these utterances can activate specific groups of muscles in the neck, the pharynx and the floor of the mouth, thus rectifying laryngeal frame asymmetries.

A few examples of the exercises designed to activate specific muscles follow:

A. For the activation of the mylohyoid muscle of the floor of the mouth he uses (with the aid of a drinking straw) the following drills with repetition of certain nonsense syllable combinations:

/jid::i: - jyd::y: - jud::u:/.

B. To rectify the dorsal resting posture of the hyoid bone, he describes the following articulatory drills with repetition of certain utterances including stressed /d/ sound:

/ji:"dn - ja:"dn - ju:"dn/,

with the apex of the tongue elevated and tucked between the maxillary incisors and the upper lip.

Selected exercises are directed toward reducing increased tension and faulty posture of the base of the tongue. Exercises are practiced daily, for 2 minutes per exercise. The patient is given no more than 3–5 exercises to be practiced at any time. Check-up is done every 2–3 weeks. Sovijarvi suggests patients require about 2-6 months for complete recovery.

Although the major bulk of this treatment program consists of vocal drills by logatomes to correct "asymmetries," it offers exercises for easing glottal "hard attack," which is considered as a manifestation of "hyperkinetic" voices. On the other hand, this method describes also some drills that may help the production of a tight voice. Sovijarvi (1984) uses in some of his exercises a drumming rhythm as a facilitatory tool.

II. FORCHHAMMER'S TECHNIQUE OF VOICE THERAPY

General Principles

Forchhammer's treatmant is based on a Gestalt philosophy; the "whole" is the sum of the components of that make up the "whole."

Thus, the integrity of the "whole" function relies on the integrity of the faulty components, and correction of dysfunctional components individually should improve the "whole." The clinician's pedagogical task, then, is to identify the defective components, and correct them individually, in order to restore the failing "whole" function.

Forchhammer defines voice production simply as an outcome of a balance between subglottic pressure and vocal fold (glottic) resistance. He maintains that diaphragmatic breathing is the most effective type of breathing for voice production, with abdominal, flank, and lumbar back muscles actively involved in the expiratory activity.

He stresses also two basic phenomena as central for healthy voice function:

1. The dynamic aspect of speaking voice as manifested by the continuous stress and tone variations.
2. The proper coordination among the different muscular components sharing in the production of voice.

Pathophysiology of Voice

Forchhammer's method of therapy is based on his concept of the pathogenesis of functional voice disorder resulting from laryngeal muscle "insufficiencies", probably due to misuse. He identifies a vocal fold adductory dysfunction resulting from "transversus" (interarytenoid) muscle insufficiency or "lateralis" (lateral cricoarytenoid) muscle insufficiency. He maintains that this type of insufficiency may lead to a posterior glottal phonatory gap and resultant inability to produce a whisper without inviting vocal fold periodic vibrations.

He describes another source of insufficiency involving the "internus" thyroarytenoid muscle or the "externus" thyroarytenoid muscle and the longitudinal tension of the vocal ligament. The imbalance between these three elements may manifest in pitch defects.

Forchhammer suggests that phonasthenia results from an increased vocal demand in the presence of an insufficient vocal mechanism that causes the patient to resort to compensatory activation of the external laryngeal muscles to "fix" (stabilize) the larynx. The static muscle contractions needed for this compensatory fixation are more exhausting than the dynamic ones. The end result of this compensatory fixation is the spread of increased tension and later pain to the pharynx and larynx.

The Therapy Program

The Forchhammer method of therapy stresses the importance of the cooperation between the clinician (pedagogue) and the patient (pupil). This is supposed to be enhanced by actively involving the patient as a pedagogic student in the treatment program; detailed explanation of the principles, goals, and steps of the training exercises and drills are provided at the onset of therapy. Forchhammer stresses the importance of enhancing both auditory and kinesthetic feedback control systems. He claims improved feedback is a necessary requisite to achieving the goals of the therapy program. A brief summary of the technique follows.

(1) Respiratory and Relaxation Exercises

Diaphragmatic breathing with abdominal and back muscle support is conducted for a few minutes every session. Also, serial relaxation exercises are practiced nearly every session to remove the tension from the face, forehead, jaw, and tongue muscles. Relaxation is thought to be facilitated by encouraging the patient to smile and yawn.

(2) Coordination

Coordination of jaw, tongue, and lip movements while producing a vocal sigh is initially prolonged with a soft breathy character. Later the prolonged tone is used in a more normal (tighter) vocal characteristic.

(3) Phonatory Drills

A series of phonatory drills are prescribed to correct the specific laryngeal muscle "insufficiencies" identified by the clinician. Many of these drills, which tend to be static and segmental, aim at enhancing the phonatory adductory activities, thus decreasing phonatory glottal waste (gap). Increasing adduction also runs the risk of producing a hard glottal attack. The clinician carefully guides the patient through this treacherous passage of balancing forces where increased adductory action without excessive force is achieved. Forchhammer describes a series of exercises with gliding tones to help reach this goal and correct certain "insufficiencies."

Forchhammer uses some facilitatory techniques. These include finger manipulation of the larynx to help correcting the "insufficiencies." He relies heavily on the use of a vibrator over the thyroid cartilage to help, as he claims, the patient to overcome the "insufficiency" in question.

(4) Articulation

This method of voice therapy claims that articulatory drills may generalize to improve vocal function. For the Accent Method (AM) and other techniques discussed in this book, articulation therapy is most logically applied during the final stages of therapy to augment vocal training by aiding in transfer of the new vocal behavior to connected speech.

REFERENCES

Forchhammer, E. (1974). *Stemmens Funktioner og fejl funktioner.* Copenhagen, Denmark: Munksgaard.

Sovijarvi, A. (1974). *Therapeutic results of laryngeal asymmetric postures in dysphonic patients.* Tokyo: World Papers in Phonetics.

Sovijarvi, A. (1984). Some therapeutic exercises for rehabilitating functional dysphonias presented on videotape. In *The study of sounds, the proceedings of the Fourth World Congress of Phoneticians,* (Vol. XX) (pp. 445–457). Japan: The Phonetic Society of Japan.

INDEX